What people are saying AFTER *Cleaning Up!*...

I lost 20 pounds in three weeks. I'm now upgrading my diet and adopting a vegetarian diet.

I'm off my ADD meds and have much clearer thoughts. I have much more energy and no longer "need" coffee in the morning. I quit smoking and can't believe the sludge that keeps pouring out of me. My boyfriend has been cleansing too, and he feels a lot calmer and more relaxed afterward.

I'm making great progress breaking up a solid lump in my shoulder—it's amazing the candida and filth that's in there. I'm 43 and feel 21. After years of neck problems and stiff joints, I'm as nimble as I was as a teenager—and I know now that stiff joints are just toxins! While I still have occasional headaches, I'm no longer having debilitating migraines. I feel very empowered to know that I can cure myself.

After cleansing two and a half months, I've lost the 15 pounds I've been struggling to lose for the last five years. More importantly, the brain fog and severe memory issues that have plagued me for years have almost completely cleared and my mental functioning seems to improve with each passing day. Thanks for the incredibly life-changing information you've published in this book.

My friend in his 70's is also doing the cleanse. He's lost 20 extra pounds, and his long-time sinus problem improved immediately. His blood pressure is also slowly coming down and a pain in his shoulder went away completely.

I've been cleansing a short time and have seen clumps of candida come out of me. The results have been fabulous...

The difference in my skin and allergies is amazing! According to blood tests, I've also cured my candida.

I was having a heart attack once a month. After following your recipe for heart problems, I haven't had a heart attack since. My doctor wants to know what I'm doing so he can tell his other patients; he's added 10 years to my life expectancy and says he's never seen anything like it.

I've done the gallbladder cleanse several times and have passed well over 100 stones. After about six months on the cleanse and also doing the gallbladder cleanse several times, I passed several cups of white gelatinous matter after doing the gallbladder cleanse. (From the author, to me this very much sounds like a cancer of the gallbladder being eliminated.)

After a bunch of fasting, colon and liver cleansing, I'm written up in a medical journal as the only person in the world with AIDS and a functioning immune system. My doctors think it's a new breed of AIDS, but I think it's the cleansing you helped me do.**

For years I've been putting up with tight hips, glutes and hamstrings. I'm just about through stage 2 of the cleanse and have had some interesting results. I've been into martial arts and yoga for 8-9 years and have only managed to get the splits and keep them for very brief amounts of time. One evening, after starting the coffee enemas, I decided to stretch without any real warm up and I gained inches when doing front and side splits. It's usually been very painful in my groin and outer hip but on this occasion, there was next to no pain and I was less than a half inch off the ground. I let it go as a one off experience and then tried again a couple of days later—and had the same results. I don't know how it worked, but I'm definitely putting it down to the cleanse.

I cleansed for three weeks and a skin problem I've had for years is 80% gone. I also added some enzyme supplements to my cleanse.

I've cleansed for just two weeks and wonderful things have happened. For one, my longtime acne is gone...

My Experience...

With some deep and aggressive cleansing, I, personally, have gotten rid of chronic insomnia, regular chest pains, chronic exhaustion, and large, rock-hard lumps along my spine, and in my throat and shoulders. I'm quite certain these lumps, or large pockets of waste, would have been called cancers or tumors, had I had them diagnosed.

I also got rid of massive candida overgrowth (literally head to toe), more toxicity than anyone would reasonably believe was in there, gallstones (a couple dozen larger ones, and thousands of mini sand-like ones), and back problems—including several areas of chronic pain and bone misalignment. The chronic hip pain and misalignment disappeared the day I passed about a foot of mucoid plaque. I eliminated an irrational fear with the passage of that plague too.

I then got rid of what was called an allergy, sinus problems, several female issues, an extreme visual sensitivity to sunlight (sunlight would hurt my eyes), and deteriorating vision. My vision still isn't perfect, but I no longer can tell it's deteriorating. According to a chiropractor, who I used to need weekly for pain, I've become less arthritic too. This statement was made early in my cleansing and I'm guessing by this point I'm not at all arthritic—but even some basic cleansing was enough for him to notice a difference.

I've also said goodbye to athlete's foot, and a brain fog that would have probably progressed into something called some sort of early onset Alzheimer's—especially if I let it continue. Years ago, my toxicity state was such that I was having trouble remembering recent events. Fortunately, that was rather easy to get rid of and bring my memory and thinking back into clarity and sharpness.

The spiritual differences I've experienced with deep cleansing aren't really explicable, so let's just say that it's a completely different experience than what I experienced pre-cleansing and on a far more normal diet. I've also had huge improvements in emotional stature and am now often handle even formerly difficult situations with ease. I've also gotten rid of several emotional blocks that were translated into behavioral blocks, serving only to hold me back. When the emotional blocks were eliminated, the behavior effortlessly changed as well. Cleansing also helped me lose about 35 extra pounds and most people who met me these days think I'm at least twelve to fifteen years younger than I am.

So, what will YOU be saying after Cleaning Up!?

As a note, I occasionally update this book to answer common questions and I've also recently tweaked the cleanse to make it easier to do and maintain, yet more powerful and more gentle. The cleansing experiences on the previous pages are from people using a slightly different version of the cleanse than the one that's in front of you. A few of these folks also benefited from using some of the information in this book, without doing the entire cleanse, and I may have also helped them individually as opposed to through this book. **In addition to the fasting, colon and liver cleansing, he also used colon cleansing pills and bentonite clay.

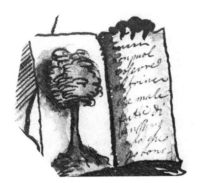

*This book is dedicated to our Higher Power,
which I believe inspired it, gave me the
information and people I needed to complete it
and put me on my path to make this information
available to the general public.
With love...*

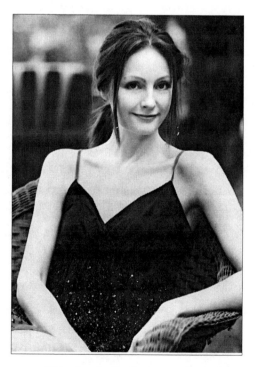

Kim Evans, or Kimberly Jo Evans - at 36 years young.

Acknowledgments

I am extraordinarily grateful to the healers who have come before me and influenced me: Dr. Richard Anderson, Steve Meyerowitz, Donna Gates, Bruce Fife, Dr. Tullio Simoncini, Dr. Stanley Bass, Dr. Alexander Ferenczi, Dr. Robert O. Young and Dr. Gabriel Cousens have all in one way or another lent their wisdom to this book. There also dozens of other authors and probably close to a hundred thousand Internet pages that I've learned from as well, and I'm truly grateful that researching natural health methods on the Internet is so accessible these days. If it were not, this book never would have contained all of the information that it does.

I'm also grateful for the wonderful people I've met on this path, who lent me books and turned me on to information that I may have used outright or tweaked in my own way to make work, as well as for the many others who have supported me and offered invaluable help and assistance along the way. Special thanks to: Lynn, Paige, Jasmine, Daniel, Tenley, Troy, Keith, James, Jo-anne, Giselle, Amy, Suzanne, and Danny. You all have my heart-felt thank you.

Thanks also to Lou Corona for adding key pieces to my theory of Adam and Eve's fall from grace, and for making sure I understood that it was living foods, not just raw foods. And thanks to Piter Caizer, who's also known as the Wheatgrass or Wildgrass Messiah, for turning me onto wild grasses and making sure I received other pertinent information along this journey. Actually, Piter sent me the e-mail that lead me to find the images from Nostradamus, and a few days later told me about the Revelation prophecy too.

More thanks to Mike Adams of Naturalnews.com, where I wrote extensively about natural health in 2009 and 2010, for helping reach people with this message—and for his tremendous work warning people about the dangers of chemical-based health care.

Another thank you to the early adopters of this cleanse whose questions and feedback while cleansing helped me refine a few viewpoints and clarify a few processes—as well as make the process more powerful, yet easier to do and maintain. I'm grateful because future cleansers, like yourself, will now benefit from a better cleanse and a book that answers more common questions—before they come up.

Last but not least, I'm grateful to my parents, who each in their own way, made sure I was loved, provided for, and well educated. They also made sure I exposed to critical thinking, storytelling, what it takes to go the extra mile, compassion, fun, and humor—while especially at a young age exposing me to endless opportunities and giving me the freedom to be creative, sometimes messy, and who I am. Without many of these things, I'm quite sure this work never would have been accomplished.

Important Note

Cleaning Up!, and *The Cleaning Up! Cleanse*, are the beliefs and suggestions of the author and therefore the sharing of this information is protected by the First Amendment to the United States Constitution.

This information is certainly not intended to replace the advice of a competent health care provider and it's always best to consult with one before embarking on a cleansing program, using supplements, or making major changes to your diet. Please don't mistake this information for medical advice—the author of this book is neither a physician nor engaged in rendering medical services to the reader. All techniques offered and recommendations given are the beliefs, suggestions, and opinions of the author and nothing more.

All information is provided with the understanding that any and all participation is at your own risk. If you don't fully accept this responsibility, please don't adopt any of these ideas or suggestions. If you have questions about your health with this program or otherwise, please consult a competent health care provider.

In any case, in no event will the author, publisher, or The Cleaning Up! Cleanse, LLC, be liable or responsible for any damage or injury caused, directly or indirectly, from any application of the information or techniques presented in *Cleaning Up!*, or from any related products or materials.

Table of Contents

The Nostradamus Prophecy

In 2007, The History Channel did an exposé on the images of the Lost Book of Nostradamus and in it, it was explained that image 67 tells us that the secrets of the Garden of Eden would be shared at a critical juncture in history. *Cleaning Up!*, even when originally published, contained this information, although, it's a little more built out in the version in front of you. Yet, I didn't come across Nostradamus' images, prophecy or The History Channel segment until February of 2011. Image 67 is also the image that Nostradamus shows someone who looks just like me, writing the book on what appears to be a laptop. You can watch some of this segment online at www.youtube.com/watch?v=Wb35IQiMdNk&NR=1 and I encourage you to check it out for some background on these images.

I wish had better quality images of Nostradamus' drawings to share with you, but for the most part they aren't accessible. My portrait and images 67 and 72 are in a few pages and I encourage you to take a minute and compare my profile to image 67. I also have better quality images at www.CleaningUpCleanse.com/Nostradamus. Alternatively, just Google "Lost book" and "image 67." Or "image 67" and "one male" to find an enlarged book to read the text, where my middle name, Jo, is the first word of the last sentence and Ron Paul's name is on the second line. In any case, upon learning that the book in his drawing contained the words "one male" it set me off to look for other recognizable words, which is when I found my first name in the wheel and my middle name in the book, as well as Ron Paul's name. My portrait, I recognized instantly.

Due to image quality, my first name is harder to read, but if you blow up the wheel a little (you can do this with images online), you'll see that the first two letters are K and y, and the third letter appears to be an N. Kyn would be pronounced Kin, similarly to how "gym" is pronounced Jim. However, from some angles, the right slant of the "y" appears to become part of the "n", making it an "m". You can see Kim in the wheel, somewhat clearly, at 1:55 and 1:56 seconds, in the video link on the previous page, but you'll need to stop the video and look closely. Either way, Nostradamus is known for misspelling names, probably in part to let history unfold as it's meant to.

Even more interesting is that there appears to be stubble on the face Nostradamus has writing the book. However, this was an area I had an extremely hard to get rid of candida problem. I had to break up and remove solid lumps in my throat and shoulders to get all of it, and since I didn't have the methods in *this* book when I started, it took forever. In any case, the area that he shows stubble, the left side of my face, would flare up each time I ate something off the candida diet. This was actually how I was able to test many foods for candida, along with using more general recommendations. I find it interesting because apparently, not only could Nostradamus look through time to see who was writing this book, he could also see through my skin and see tremendous amounts of toxic filth. It certainly validates what they say: nothing in this world is hidden...

I've actually been aware for years that the book I've been writing was prophesied and of the power of the information contained within it. However, it wasn't until early 2011 that I learned *where* it was prophesied or had any evidence to show people so, for the most part, I just kept it to myself. You should also know that I'm very much a normal person. Granted, a normal person who's now extremely clean and with a different diet, but human, nonetheless. So, I'm just the messenger... The real magic is in this book, and specifically when the information in this book is applied. And it'll be ridiculously powerful when it's applied in massive ways and we're living in clean bodies and chemical-free, love-centered, raw food communities again. Actually, it'll be ridiculously powerful if 1 percent of the population gravitates to it and becomes spiritually connected again.

A lot of people are uncertain what this time in history means, so here's what I know. It's my understanding that at this time we can light a fire of consciousness across the planet that will be unstoppable and will dispel the darkness that's becoming so evident all around us. However, it'll require that millions of people cleanse deeply and follow the other dietary guidance in this book to bring about this powerful energy and consciousness shift. So, I hope you're all up for the journey—because the final outcome is not assured, but rather up for humankind to choose by their actions.

In image 72, which is on the next page, Nostradamus shows the book being delivered—and scholars tell us this is right around 2012. The lamb in the bottom of this image tells us that this book also is the Book of Life in Revelation, which is prophesied to be delivered by the lamb. Oddly, I was born in year 1972. Of course, the lamb's Book of Life is the book that the *Bible* says brings people to enlightenment.

It's widely interpreted that Jesus is the lamb of the Revelation prophecy, however, in John 1:29 - 30, Jesus tells us that he is not. The *Bible* in front of me reads, "Look, the Lamb of God, who takes away the sin of the world! This is the one I meant when I said, 'A man who comes after me has surpassed me because he was before me. I myself did not know him, but the reason I came baptizing with water was that he might be revealed to Israel.'"

Of course, different versions use different words, but the message is clear that Jesus is not the lamb, and also that the reason he was here a few thousand years back was to prepare the way for someone else.

Actually, if you look at the Essene *Gospel of Peace* (www.essene. com/GospelOfPeace/peace1.html) which gets into many of Jesus' holistic teachings, you'll see that a good deal of what he was teaching was about cleansing, raw foods, and natural living—as a path to higher consciousness. If you read his words in the *Bible* with this understanding, what he was saying actually makes a lot more sense.

One example is Revelation 22: 14, "Blessed are those who wash their robes, that they might have the right to the tree of life." The robes are our bodies, or the clothing for our soul. Of course, the tree of life is depicted in Nostradamus' image 67 in the book and it's a reference to the spiritual connection that I speak of. John 6:27 also get right to the heart of the matter, "Do not work for food that spoils, but for food that endures to eternal life, which the Son of Man will give you. On him God the Father has placed his seal of approval." It's hard to say that God the Father has placed his seal on anything but unaltered foods from nature. Matthew 23:26 also makes a lot more sense if you understand he's talking about cleansing, "First clean the inside of the cup and then the outside also will be clean." This is from the famous passage where he's calling the Pharisees hypocrites.

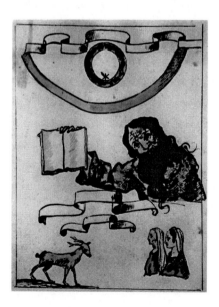

My Portrait...

This picture was taken in February 2011 about two weeks after my 39th birthday. I took it of myself the day I found Nostradamus' image 67 to compare my profile to his image. In truth, I never expected to share this picture with anyone and it was taken a day or two before I found the Revelation prophecy—or knew anything about a lamb or someone coming under a rainbow to deliver a prophesied book. In any case, I wore this rainbow scarf daily for about two weeks before and after this picture was taken. It is (or was...) a scarf of my mom's, and I picked it up one night, wrapped it around my head, and sort of formed an attachment to it. I also found that energy was directed to my crown chakra when wearing it, which was quite powerful. You can see the color image online at www.CleaningUpCleanse.com/Nostradamus.

About a month later, when I was getting ready to send *Cleaning Up!* to the printer, I planned to take a better photo, one where my hair was done and I'd made an effort to look decent, but the Universe let me know that this was picture to use. So, even though it's far from the best picture I've seen of myself, this is the one I'll share.

The image is unretouched and has only been resized. You can probably see that on my left cheek, I had a mole there once. I removed it years ago with some herbal cream that I bought online and I bring this up because in the previous section, I talk about how I had a big candida and toxicity problem in this area—and later in this book, I share how dark moles are often markers of large amounts of filth—which interestingly, made it into Nostradamus' drawing, as what appears as stubble.

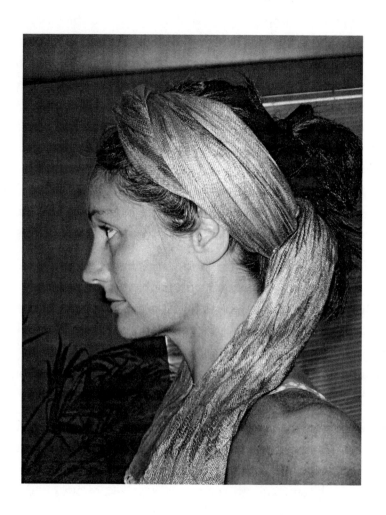

Revelation Prophecy...

I think my favorite line in Relevation is 22:4, "They will see his face, and his name will be on their foreheads." This is the passage that then talks about humans living by the light. As odd as it seems, I'm apparently supposed to be sharing these images with you at this time and revealing my identity as the author of the Book of Life, and even me sharing it in this way was predestined. Of course, I didn't find this line until after I'd found these images and had planned to make this information publicly available. This line gives me comfort because making such an announcement about yourself is a very strange thing to be doing and the obvious thought is, "What if people don't believe it?" But, as I explain later in *Cleaning Up!*, on their foreheads is just another way of saying that people will believe it.

So, if you pull out any Bible (and I encourage you to do so), and compare Nostradamus' images with the Revelation prophecy, you'll see that all he's doing in images 66-72 is drawing parts of the Revelation prophecy. You can see the complete book from Nostradamus here: www.youtube.com/watch?v=MnAwK2Li77Q. Just stop and pause on any images you like, and if you do so while reading this section, what I'm saying will probably make a lot more sense.

So, let's go over the seven end of time images. The first image, image 66, is the lion and if you read Revelation 22:16 *and* 5:4-6, you'll see that Jesus is the loin (but not the lamb). In this image, he'll see him basking in the sun, and the sun is representative of our higher power. The star of David is also in this image, and in Rev 22:16 Jesus calls himself "the offspring of David and the bright morning star."

In image 67, Nostradamus shows us the woman who comes with the crown on her head that's talked about in Revelation 12. This, of course, is also the image that looks just like me and as I've described, you can find my name in it. Revelation 12:5 talks about this

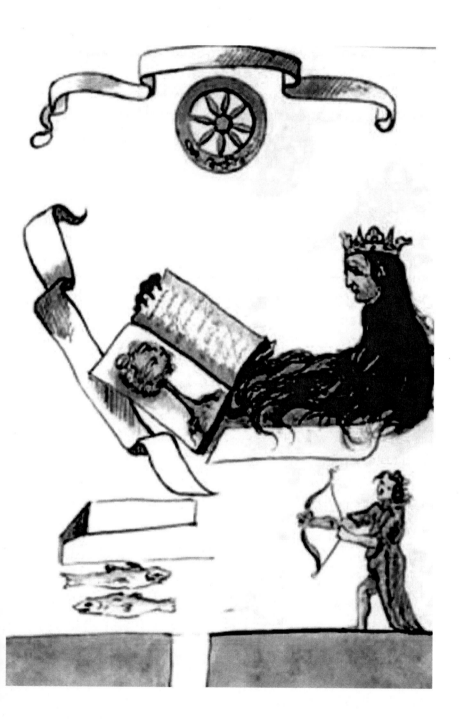

woman giving birth to a male son who is meant to "rule all nations with an iron scepter." All I can really tell you is that *Cleaning Up!* has always had a blue cover, long before I learned of this prophecy. This book was also written in my child bearing years, and most certainly, in lieu of having children. In fact, when I was just barely into cleansing, I was guided in a mediation, telling me I wasn't meant to have any children. Of course, at the time, I had no idea why but I understood that I was hearing the voice of our higher power, so I just accepted it.

Nostradamus uses also scrolls in his seven "end of time" images and scrolls are talked about in Revelation too. In fact, the scroll is called the *book* in some *Bible* translations. In some of the images, I believe the scrolls are also a reference to the uploading and downloading of information on the Internet and also to the spiritual connection I speak of in this book.

In Revelation 10, it talks about an angel with a rainbow over his head, who comes down to deliver the scroll (or the book). Actually, I find it a bit funny because Revelation 10:9 reads, "So I went to the angel and asked him to give me the little scroll. He said to me, 'Take it and eat it. It will turn your stomach sour, but in your mouth it will taste like honey.'" I find this funny because obviously, it's a book about food, and well, turning your stomach sour, is a way of saying that some people really won't like the news. But on the bright side, at least it implies you'll like my recipes.

Anyway, the character with the bow in image 67, I believe is my friend, Piter Caizer, who as I mentioned earlier, sent me the e-mail that lead me to find Nostradamus' images. Then, a few days later he directed me to the Revelation prophecy. If you look him up online, you'll see it looks just like him, and you can find him by the names the Wheatgrass Messiah or Wildgrass Messiah. You may also find that he dresses a bit on the feminine side, which has lead many people to believe this character is a female.

In any case, the words 'one male' in the text of Nostradamus' book, I believe refers to the e-mail he sent. If he had not, I'm sure I wouldn't have so much of your attention right now, which as I understand it, was the reason for the prophecies in the first place. Revelation also refers to someone with a bow, who's fighting back some evil that is coming. However, as I understand it, this only comes if we don't make the consciousness shift that I referred to earlier and it can be averted.

A lot of people think this evil is coming in 2012, but I don't. I think that's the time the energy will be read on the planet and it will be determined which prophecy will come to pass. The one with humans living in the light, or the other that Nostradamus talks of, with the Antichrist leading the way. If the later comes to pass, it'll will make the darkness that's all around us these days look like a day at the beach. And is that really a fair gift to our children?

The next image, 68, shows a face off between the lamb and scorpion, or what's really a fight between good and evil. Of course, both the lamb and scorpion are referred to in Revelation and it's pretty clear who's on the side of good and who's on the side of evil. The scorpions are also referred to as locusts. In Nostradamus' image, there's also a scroll that's depicted taking down a human held sword. Of course, the sword is a reference to the violence and control that's all around us.

Below the lamb and scorpion is a book and above them, we can see that the Tree of Life, referenced in Revelation and drawn in the book in image 67, has been impinged upon by what one scholar calls "some monster." The Tree of Life is really higher consciousness, or enlightenment, and the life experiences that are available when you live there. Of course, I've done my best to write the path there, here, in this book.

In image 69 we see a blindfolded man pointing his bow and arrow at a woman. I actually believe this refers to an incident in my life in February 2011, when I tried to share this information with my friend Piter, including my role in it, and well, he already believed something different. So, like people sometimes do when you share information that's different than what they believe, he kind of attacked me (verbally) a little bit. On the bright side, from this rather negative energy exchange, I came up with the chakra clearing methods in Chapter 12, which for me, worked like a charm. And all is forgiven at this point.

Scholars tell us that image 70 is the time line, using astrology that I don't understand. However, they say it points right to 2012 and an astrological event that only happens every 13,000 years in which the sun rises in perfect alignment with the center of the galaxy. In this image, the only scroll is at the top and it's blue. The blue scroll may be a reference to the "male son" and the scroll, we've talked about, is also sometimes called a book.

Image 71, I believe, is Nostradamus holding his book and he's showing us his book, letting us know that his images would be understood at this time. There is also an Ark at the top of this image and in this way, I believe Nostradamus is telling us that understanding his images will save people, as the Ark did. Interestingly, Nostradamus predicted that his images wouldn't be understood for 500 years past his time, and 500 years ago, he was alive.

Image 72, we've talked about, is the last of Nostradamus' seven end of time images, and it shows the book being delivered, right around 2012. There's also a line below the wheel of an Ark, and I believe it's there to show that the methods in the Book of Life are the path to the light that's described in the Revelation prophecy.

If you look around with an open eye, you might see that evil has been winning the battle for sometime now, especially when you understand that chemicals and even cooked foods are the common tools to disconnect us spiritually. However, according Revelation, it's time to make a shift now. It's written in 23:3, "No longer will there be any curse. The throne of God and of the Lamb will be in the city, and his servants will serve him." It then goes on to talk about humans now living in the light for "ever and ever." The curse is obviously the curse of the Garden of Eden, and later in *Cleaning Up!*, it explains how we got there.

So... When I was growing up, my Dad used to say, "You can either be part of the problem or part of the solution." He also once said, "Before you knew the truth, you had an excuse, but now that you know the truth, you don't have that excuse any more." So, the question becomes, now that you know, how will you choose?

Interestingly, the Japanese quake was also the quake in Revelation 16:17-19. I'm sure of this because I wrote e-mail as the quake was happening, literally real time, saying, "I think I finally got this book done." Actually, it was to a person at the Environmental Working Group, who I'd met the evening before. I promised to send her some information the next day, and it was getting late, so I did. In this passage it says, "The seventh angel poured out his bowl into the air and out of the temple came a loud voice from the throne, saying "It is done!" Then came flashes of lighting, rumblings, peals of thunder and a severe earthquake. No earthquake like it has ever occurred since man has been on earth, so tremendous was the quake." Of course, I didn't read this passage until the next day and according to my e-mail, I pushed send about three minutes after the quake started. Obviously, this was before the Tsunami or anyone realized how bad it was going to get.

I think the Japanese quake is also the dragon referred to in Revelation 12, which happens right as the woman is about to give birth. Dragons are symbolic of Japan and this passage talks of a serpent spewing water from his mouth, or the Tsunami. Even as this book is heading to the printer, they still haven't gotten it under control and in the news of today, March 30th, it appears it's getting worse. As it turns out, this book wasn't really done on March 10th (California time), it took me another few weeks to finish it. But that's the way my world works—what the Universe has in store for me next, I very often have no idea.

In any case, *Cleaning Up!* was updated with new techniques and information, and this final version will be available in April 2011. It took me almost seven years of unwavering commitment, but I think I finally have all of the information in this book that's meant to be here.

Now, as the Universe has guided and because I really would love to see a massive, positive energy and consciousness shift on the planet, where enlightenment becomes the norm instead of a rarity, I'm making *Cleaning Up!* available as a free e-book to anyone who would like a copy. Of course, you're welcome to e-mail this book to friends and family, so long as it's without charging or making any changes. It's also allowable to post the PDF on websites for free download, so long as nothing is added or subtracted, or any changes made. Making print copies of the book, however, isn't allowable as it may interfere with future distribution that I need to set up. In any case, I'm guided at this time to make *Cleaning Up!* as widely available as possible, so help with this is very much appreciated. You can also send to people to my Website to grab a copy there, and in doing so, they'll start receiving my newsletter too.

If you'd like to support this project and help bring this information freely into the world in the scale that it's intended, donations are warmly accepted and can be done at www.CleaningUpCleanse.com. Of course, if you're cleansing, purchasing your supplies from the site helps me out too. I wrote this book and developed these methods on a dime and a shoestring, so it's more appreciated than you know.

More Peaceworkers

Other organizations that are doing great work and could also use financial funding are:

Natural Solutions Foundation: they are on the front lines of fighting some of the worst of what's happening to our food supply and the poisons that are often in vaccines, etc.

www.healthfreedomusa.org

Environmental Working Group: they test for numerous toxic substances in our bodies (and regularly find them!). They also test consumer products and work on governmental levels to get consumer protection built into the equation (because right now it rarely is), while educating consumers about them as well.

www.ewg.org

The Institute for Responsible Technology: they are the strongest force around fighting GMOs and they do great work to educate consumers about them too.

www.responsibletechnology.org

News...

If you want to get in touch with what's happening to our food supply, and other great holistic health news, I strongly recommend free e-mail subscriptions to www.naturalnews.com or www.mercola.com. Both will do a good job of getting you up to speed with important information that doesn't always make the mainstream press. Dr. Steve also does a wonderful radio program on www.healthylife.net Wednesdays at 1pm PT and archives of his shows are available too.

Chapter 1

The Average Person

Congratulations for picking up this book. With that simple step, you're well on your way to making one of the most dramatic, positive changes in your life you can imagine. Eliminating massive amounts of toxicity from the body can and regularly does result in the elimination of health problems and excess weight—while also providing a deeper spiritual connection to our divine source. Actually, since eliminating toxicity so regularly brings these positive things, then you must understand that it was the accumulation of toxicity that brought the negative side—ill health, disconnection from our divine source, and excess weight—in the first place. But let's start by looking at where we are...

The average person carries an extreme toxic burden and most of the time, is completely unaware of it. I sometimes wonder if even people would think they were healthy if our skin were see-if through—because we'd see a completely different picture. So, let's start by looking at some of the causes.

The average person eats non-organic foods regularly, which means he or she is consuming small amounts of pesticides and herbicides each day. Pesticides and herbicides are designed to kill living organisms. So, do you really think the daily ingestion of substances made for killing won't create any problems, or have any effects whatsoever?

The average person consumes processed foods each day—which contain a huge mix of often unpronounceable chemicals. The average person also eats his or her weight in food coloring and preservatives each year. Do you think our bodies can eliminate all of these chemicals on a regular basis?

The average person regularly and unknowingly eats genetically modified foods. This means, for example, that a scientist has tweaked the genes of an ear of corn so that the corn now *grows its own pesticides* continuously—yet left it looking like a normal ear of corn. Do you think it's okay that we're eating these strange inventions, or that they won't cause long-term harm?

The average person adds to their burden with regular sugar and alcohol consumption. Some people add to their burden even further with cigarettes and chemically derived drugs—especially those from a doctor. Do you really think we can eliminate all of this—day in and day out—without any excess accumulation in the body? Did you know that "properly prescribed" pharmaceuticals are the third leading killer in the U.S.?

The average person eats animals that have been treated with hormones and antibiotics—which are passed on to the people who consume these animals and drink their milk. Do you think you need these extra hormones and antibiotics? Do you know that antibiotics destroy the foundation of the human immune system? Did you know that non-organic chickens are often fed arsenic?

The average person takes in fluoride and chlorine each day through the water supply, which can enter your body through your mouth or your skin. Do you know that fluoride has been used to placate prisoners and is the sole ingredient in many rat poisons? Did you know that chlorine was used as a weapon in world war one?

The average person is exposed to pesticides in the garden and has regular contact with "normal" household cleaning supplies. Do you think these substances with danger labels won't affect you? Did you know that when scientists look, they regularly find these chemicals in even the blood of newborns?

The average person regularly breaths in fumes from automobiles—along with a disturbing amount of metals, molds, and chemicals in the environment. The average person also has mercury, one of the most brain damaging metals known, sitting inches from their brain and leaking from the metal fillings in his or her teeth. If white fillings were used, that person would have excess estrogen being released, contributing to hormonal issues. What effect do you think these substances are having on you?

The average person lives unaware of a fungal overgrowth growing in his or her body, and caused in large part by antibiotics, processed foods, and excess sugar consumption.

This fungal overgrowth, called candida overgrowth, releases more than *eighty* toxic by-products each and every day. Do you think those toxic by-products might have any effect on your emotions and health?

The average person is exposed to a great deal of radiation from cell phones, wireless Internet connections, and medical tests. Radiation is well known to cause cancer, so do you think it might have an effect on the cells of your body? How often do you hold a cell phone next to your head? How often do you hold your laptop on your lap?

The average person has ten or more pounds of old fecal matter encrusted upon his or her colon walls—and some of it may have been there since childhood. How dramatically do you think this impacts a person's health and vitality?

Women especially have the excess burden of chemicals from lotions and cosmetics because 90 percent of what's applied to the skin ends up in the bloodstream. Have you looked recently at the chemicals you're applying to your skin, or really, adding to your bloodstream?

If you want to really shock yourself, I encourage you to make a list of the chemical ingredients in your foods, lotions, cosmetics, shampoos, and soaps—everything you put in or on your body, for one week. Just look at the ingredients and write down all of the chemicals involved. For each non-organic meal, make sure you leave a few placeholders for unknown chemicals and pesticides. At the end of one week, the average person will have a list of several hundred chemicals,

Common Toxins in the Body

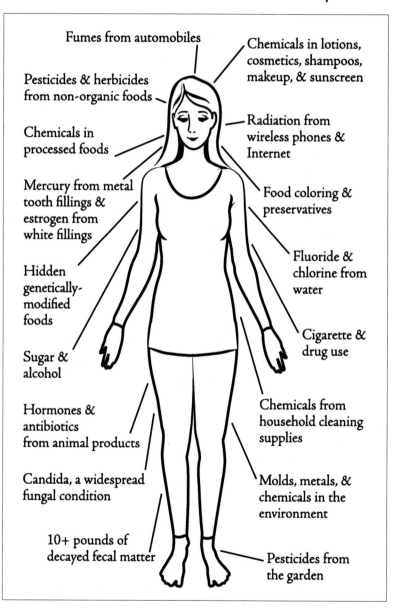

Fumes from automobiles

Chemicals in lotions, cosmetics, shampoos, makeup, & sunscreen

Pesticides & herbicides from non-organic foods

Chemicals in processed foods

Radiation from wireless phones & Internet

Mercury from metal tooth fillings & estrogen from white fillings

Food coloring & preservatives

Hidden genetically-modified foods

Fluoride & chlorine from water

Sugar & alcohol

Cigarette & drug use

Hormones & antibiotics from animal products

Chemicals from household cleaning supplies

Candida, a widespread fungal condition

Molds, metals, & chemicals in the environment

10+ pounds of decayed fecal matter

Pesticides from the garden

most of which were nonexistent on the planet just a hundred years ago. Yet, this list won't even include the chemicals we're exposed to daily from carpets, plastics, paints, and other common sources—which scientists regularly find in the blood of newborns too.[1]

The next step is to simply multiply the number of chemicals on your list by the number of weeks you've been alive, and at some point you might begin to understand how much toxicity is really in your body. Of course, your body does eliminate toxins each day as part of its normal routine, but our bodies just weren't designed for what we call "normal" living these days. In fact, in terms of human evolution, normal living and eating today, aren't at all normal. It's also key to remember that if your body can't eliminate those toxins because your detoxification systems are overwhelmed, your body has no choice but to store these poisons. Actually, stored toxins explain why health, weight, emotional, and spiritual problems are so evident in individuals of all ages. And it's what I hope to address by making this information available to you.

But, humor me for a second if you will. Think back to your high school chemistry class. You might remember that it's the *combination* of chemicals that makes them all the more

---

1   To really understand how toxic all these chemicals are to us, I encourage you to read *Detoxify or Die* by Dr. Sherry A. Rogers. She clearly spells out the highly toxic, yet common, ingredients in our foods and everyday living and points to a number of studies too. Dr. Rogers also points out that many "everyday" chemicals easily induce cancer and other serious problems in animals. You can also look at the testing of umbilical cord blood done by the Environmental Working Group. When you see all of the chemicals they find, know they're only testing for about half of one percent of all of the chemicals in use: http://www.ewg.org/reports/bodyburden2/execsumm.php.

dangerous. So, I ask you: What in the world is going on in your body? Do you think this combination of trapped chemicals and toxins could be the reason so many people have health problems today? Do you think it might be part of the reason that almost one in a hundred infants are now born with autism related disorders? Here's the real question: Do you want to get those chemicals and toxins *out* of your body to improve your health, well being and spiritual connectedness? You'll also be doing an enormous favor to any children you may have.

So, to help you answer, let me ask you a few questions.

- Do you think a body free of chemicals and toxins would have better health? Or do you think we're healthier drowning in chemical poisons?
- Do you think such a body would have better energy?
- Do you think that a toxin-free body would feel better emotionally? (Before you answer, remember that each of us is a contained system—and the brain and nervous system are never more than a few feet from any toxins stored in the body.)
- I neither make—nor intend to make—any comments about anyone's religion or spirituality, but if you believe we can be connected to the divine source of the universe (whatever name you call that source), do you think you might have a better shot at attaining that connection if you lived in a body free of chemical and toxic waste?

✺ Do you think it's possible that the toxicity in your body *could* be at the root of your problems—whether they are physical, mental, emotional, or spiritual?

✺ And how will you feel once you've succeeded in removing those problems from your body and your life? How much would that add to your life?

✺ Importantly, what consequences are you likely to suffer if you don't address these problems? Besides you, who else will it affect?

So, now for the most important question:

✺ Do you think it's about time you removed all those years' accumulation of toxicity? If so, this book will guide you through the hows and whys, making sure you under stand each step of one of the most effective, comprehen-sive, and hopefully, easy-to-do cleanses ever created.

If you need motivation during your cleanse, just come back to this page and review your answers.

Chapter 2

So, *What Does The Cleaning Up! Cleanse™ Do?*

The Cleaning Up! Cleanse is designed to thoroughly, powerfully, and painlessly detoxify your entire body. It's done by removing massive amounts of accumulated waste from your system, all of which the average person carries around regardless of whether he or she is aware of it. Why is this important? More often than not, deep cleansing eliminates health issues and prevents future problems. Lessened toxicity also plays a key role in enhancing well-being and your quality of energy.

The truth is: we're living in a society where health problems, large and small, are the norm. Yet very little connection is made between how we treat our bodies, how we have treated them over the years, and the health problems we produce as a result.

The average person doesn't understand the direct connection between the accumulated "junk" in his or her system and the symptoms he or she is experiencing. Generally, people don't recognize that excess sugar and a poor diet can cause far more serious consequences than weight problems. They also don't know that much of what people put in and on their bodies is actually harmful. Even what most people think of as healthy leaves *a lot* to be desired.

The average person also doesn't appreciate that our bodies aren't designed for the regular dousing of chemicals from processed foods, lotions, pesticides, preservatives, and all of the other chemicals that most people take in daily. Yet, because our bodies aren't designed to handle these poisons, we can't effectively eliminate them—and what we can't eliminate, *we store*. And when we store enough, we become sick. Actually, many diseases are just a reflection of where those toxins are stored, which poisons they are, and how much of them is in there.

In addition, when a body has too much toxicity to handle, it will start packing it away throughout the body, and eventually form hard lumps, or what I call pockets of waste. These pockets of waste are the body's way of containing the filth, often with clumps of candida, that it was unable to eliminate. Your body does this as an attempt to keep those poisons from constantly circulating in your blood. However, eventually these lumps, or toxicity sites, cause problems too—and if a doctor finds one, it certainly won't be a diagnosis you'd be happy to receive.

Actually, stored toxins are also the reason we identify many health problems with aging. However, most problems attributed to aging have little to do with getting older. They have far more to do with the fact that older individuals have been accumulating these toxins longer—and their bodies are losing the ability to cope. Today, it's becoming more and more common to see problems that used to be attributed to aging, in young people. This is due to considerably more toxic foods and lifestyles, which are often highly chemical in nature, and unfortunately, so common today. Today, diseases that used to take 60 or 70 years of toxic exposure to create are often being developed in 20 or 30 years.

Truthfully, when you understand the amount of toxicity the average person carries, the reason we have so many health problems as a society should become obvious. Actually, it's all pretty logical too.

It makes sense that accumulated waste in the body would affect how the body operates. It's clear that poisons in and near the nervous system would affect our emotions and our ability to handle stress. It's certainly understandable that accumulated toxicity in the joints and muscles would determine whether there is inflammation or pain. It's also logical that accumulated waste in or near an organ would affect its operation. However, if we don't understand the connection, we might assume we have a faulty organ. It's also reasonable that masses of accumulated waste would cause endless other minor and serious malfunctions. In fact, it's with common chemicals and poisons that scientists regularly create every disease imaginable in animals, so they can test pharmaceutical drugs on them.

Years ago, I didn't understand these connections either and culturally, we're not taught to recognize them. In fact, most of us are taught to poison ourselves instead. For me, it wasn't until I did a deep cleanse while in Southeast Asia that I began to understand the power of cleansing. As a result of that cleanse, I immediately let go of two chronic health problems and really, my eyes flew wide open. So, for what ended up being almost seven years afterward, I spent literally thousands of hours researching, studying, cleansing, and experimenting with different cleansing techniques. Of course, that immersive experience ultimately lead to the development of this cleanse and the cleansing techniques in this book.

All together, cleansing helped me eliminate over a dozen problems in my own body, including five that doctors had no solutions for. Of course, their only solution was drugs, if I was willing to take them. But when I saw how quickly cleansing worked for problems doctors couldn't figure out, their drugs became a humorous solution for me.

For me, in addition to eliminating so many seemingly unrelated health problems, cleaning out my own toxicity also brought me a significantly higher *quality* of energy, which changed my life.[2] Actually, when you understand that like

---

2   To learn how life events and different levels of consciousness are related to our energetic states, check out David Hawkins' book, *Power Vs. Force*. It's a heady read, but contains quite powerful information. You'll also learn how your consciousness affects everything in your life.

energy attracts like energy—it becomes obvious how elevating one's energy can dramatically improve every area of one's life.

A clean body is also a ready vehicle for the divine, if you are interested in accessing your spiritual side. I believe this has to do with the elevated energy just discussed, and the absence of toxicity to interfere with your energetic connection to our divine source. It's actually common for people carrying even light toxic burdens to experience a direct connection to our divine source, which provides a path to your higher purpose and guidance. It also leads to easily available states of contentment and bliss, and you'll likely begin experiencing plenty of divine synchronicities to guide your path and delight you along the way.

But, unfortunately, the average person carries an extreme toxic burden, even if he or she doesn't know it or denies its existence. Even newborns are born with hundreds of poisons, already in their blood. Most people also don't understand what's possible in terms of spiritual connectedness and how incredible life can be. I'd like to bring the regular states of bliss and contentment that are possible into common consciousness, to allow people to make choices based on the reality of the situation, rather than on the often limited versions of spiritual reality they've learned about so far. In any case, this book is designed to be a how to guide if you'd like to take the steps there. Or, you can just do a quick cleanse, whatever you like.

So.... What Does
The Cleaning Up! Cleanse Do?

✳ Removes enormous amounts of toxic matter from your entire body

✳ Creates an oxygen-rich alkaline internal environment in which many common problems aren't able to thrive and often can't exist

✳ Facilitates the massive removal of candida overgrowth (a pesky, common fungal problem discussed in the next section)

✳ Allows for the breaking down and removal of huge "pockets" of waste throughout the body

✳ Removes accumulated filth and hardened toxic plaque from the large and small intestines

✳ Removes bacteria, parasites, and viruses from the system

✳ Detoxifies the liver so that it can do more than a thousand jobs in the body, including detoxifying the blood and burning fat

✳ Removes heavy metals, chemicals, and radiation so they can't do the damage they are known for

✳ Cleans up the bloodstream and cleans out the sinus cavities

✳ Re-supplies the body's internal ecosystem with plenty of healthy bacteria

Chapter 3

Candida—What Is It?

It's estimated that 90 percent of the population has a problem with candida overgrowth—although most don't know
what it is or that they have a problem with it. To top it off,
this overgrowth is said to be the cause of literally *hundreds* of
different health problems. So, candida, what is it? Candida
is a yeast. In a healthy body, it's found in small amounts in
the colon, along with other healthy bacteria. Actually, present in small amounts, it has a useful function to perform:
when we die, it helps decompose our body. But, it becomes
a problem comes when candida grows from small amounts
to large proportions while we're still living. Then it morphs
into a fungus, leaves the colon and starts decomposing the
body a little too early for most people's liking. And unfortunately, this is happening in far too many bodies these days.

It's of obvious significance, but much of the medical community doesn't acknowledge candida as the cause of the
problems that bring paying customers to their offices. Of
course, there's *a lot* of money in pharmaceutical drugs, and
even well-informed doctors with the very best of intentions
are extremely limited in advising patients by what they have

been taught and by the powers that influence and control them. I bring this up because I'm sure a couple of people are wondering, "If it's such a big problem, and it's causing my symptoms, why isn't my doctor talking to me about it?" This, by the way, is an excellent question! I sincerely wish my doctors had talked to me about it, instead of leaving me on my own to figure it out. But, so it is...

Candida gets out of hand when the healthy bacteria in our colon are killed because it's the job of our healthy bacteria to keep down the yeast and other unfriendly bacteria populations. And without our healthy bacteria, the candida yeast and unfriendly bacteria proliferate wildly and eventually destroy our health. Candida overgrowth is also called systemic candida, candidiasis, or just candida, as I will refer to it.

Antibiotics, birth control pills, and steroids *regularly* kill the healthy bacteria in our guts that are meant to keep candida in check. Diets high in sugar, refined carbohydrates, and processed foods do the same thing. Even one dose of broad-spectrum antibiotics, unless you replenish your healthy bacteria, can set you up for problems, especially if you eat sugar or carbohydrates afterwards, as both feed candida. Antibiotics are how my problem initially grew out of hand, although I'm fairly certain I was born with a mild overgrowth situation. It's unfortunate but true that candida easily passes from mother to child in the womb.

The literal meaning of the word antibiotics is anti-life, and I'd never take them again. If I were ever in a situation where

I "needed" them, I'd cleanse and do lots of raw garlic and coconut oil instead. Antibiotics are dangerous because most are indiscriminate about which bacteria they kill. They wipe out the unfriendly bacteria you are taking them for *and* the good bacteria in your colon. Because these good bacteria form the basis of your immune system, their elimination can cause a whole host of problems—including the hundreds of different conditions of which candida is often the underlying cause.

So, it's important to replenish your healthy bacteria with probiotics after taking antibiotics, and consider taking coconut oil as an anti-fungal if you're on antibiotics. If your health care provider doesn't tell you to replenish your healthy bacteria after taking antibiotics, ask why they didn't. It's spelled out in *The Merck Manual* that using antibiotics can cause this overgrowth, yet this key information is rarely passed on to patients. Personally, I await the day when class action lawyers get involved with this; I'm guessing there's more money in it than in pharmaceuticals. But, until that time comes, women taking birth control and anyone taking steroids should also be conscientious about heartily replacing their healthy bacteria. As a society, we also need to get back to eating lots of foods from nature, and leaving behind the sugar-rich and carbohydrate-dense diets. Our own dietary choices are also very much to blame, even if antibiotics do set us up to fall.

Anyhow, let's look at how candida operates. After candida grows in the colon, it morphs into a fungus and forms roots. Then the fungus eats holes right through your colon walls, creating what the medical community calls "leaky gut syndrome." When this occurs, a number of things can and do happen next. With holes in your colon walls, waste from your colon escapes and enters your bloodstream—where it's not supposed to be—causing allergic reactions, fatigue, and other symptoms. Waste from your colon in your blood is *obviously* not a good thing—think about it for a minute. As if that weren't enough, the fungus, too, now spreads throughout your body, no longer limiting itself to your colon. The fungus gets into the muscles and tissues, where it continues to grow unchecked. It often nests in organs and severely compromises them. My own overgrowth was literally head to toe, and like most people, I had no idea that my diet was feeding it and making it worse.

Candida overgrowth can be the cause of so many problems because candida can lodge and nest in so many different areas of the body. If it lodges in your sinuses, you might have a sinus condition, allergies, or vision problems. If it nests in the muscles of your low back, you may have low back pain or bones that go out of alignment. If it's in your shoulders, you might "carry tension" in your shoulders (which will block blood flow to your brain). If the overgrowth is severe in your muscles, it might be called fibromyalgia. If it's in an organ, you might have problems with that organ, or with the functions that the organ is supposed to handle. When candida is in your skin, it looks like acne, athlete's foot, a rash, whitish spots, or eczema. If it's solid lump anywhere in your body, one oncologist who has a *far better* cancer rate than chemotherapy doctors (who lose, as a note, about half their patients), is saying it's called cancer. Of course, that oncologist (who we'll talk more about in the next chapter) has had his license stripped, which is what I mean by the powers that be that control medical doctors[3]. I, personally, have a hard time looking at pictures of things like cysts, fibroids, endometriois, or Crohn's Disease, and not seeing giant lumps of candida. I look at pictures of Alzheimer's brains and see that the "plaque" associated with the disease is candida lodged in their brain. Then, I look at pictures of things like cancers and tumors and see more large candida clumps that look like what came out of me with some very deep and aggressive cleansing. You're probably starting to see how deeply this runs.

Brain tumors, in particular, because they're not coated with blood and lymph as many other cancers are—look exactly like candida clumps. Actually, if you're curious about any disease, go to Google images and see if it involves having white or whitish yellow lumps or clumps in the body. You might need to look at several pictures, because some can be covered with a little blood and mucus but you might be very surprised at what you find.

Unfortunately, it gets worse. Candida is a living organism that releases close to eighty toxic by-products into the body, each and everyday. One of these by-products is chemically similar to formaldehyde. How do you think you'd feel after having

---

3   If the dangerous shenanigans that regularly go on in the medical world (that more often than not put profits *way* before people) are new to you, I highly recommend a free e-mail subscription from www.naturalnews.com.If you're more conservative in your views, but want to get educated on this stuff, you'd probably enjoy a free e-mail subscription from www.mercola.com. If you prefer your news in an audio format, Dr. Steve gives a great show Wednesday's at 1PT on www.healthylife.net.

something close to formaldehyde being pumped out in abundance in your body everyday? How do you think you'd think if you had all that going on in or near your brain? Of course all of the toxins released by candida can cause headaches or migraines. These toxins can even be the source of rage, anger, and depression—it's something that societies with violence problems and families with behavioral problems might want to seriously consider. In women, the effects of candida often show up as PMS, as cyclical estrogen feeds the overgrowth. It can also show itself as "brain fog" and be related to problems with memory, concentration and ADD—even in children. The list continues and unfortunately, it can be pretty long.

On top of all of the other toxic burdens we face, candida creates *a lot* of toxicity for a body to deal with. Yet, approximately nine out of ten people have candida overgrowth. So, is it any wonder that 40 percent of the U.S. population is indefinitely on pharmaceutical drugs? The reasons why should be becoming very clear.

Now, for the good news. As if by a miracle, once the overgrowth is brought under control and eliminated, many of the symptoms, once seen as disease or emotional problems, can simply vanish from the body. It seems like magic, but in reality it's understanding the source of the problem and removing it. So I ask you, if candida is the underlying cause of any health condition you or a loved one is facing, would it be better to take drugs to mask the symptoms, or to remove the problem before it spawns more problems?

Up to this point, candida has been notoriously difficult to get rid of. Even with these methods, it does take some time and effort. Candida diets slow the growth and can cause the fungus to die, but they often fail to eliminate the problem even after years of strict adherence. I followed the candida diet for well over a year before I discovered many of the protocols in this book, and the amount of candida that came out of me when I used these methods was astounding. The diet alone *never* would have eliminated my full-blown overgrowth or the pesky health problems that came along with it. Most products I've tried won't even touch a serious overgrowth situation, and they can be quite expensive.

The Cleaning Up! Cleanse is incredibly effective. It removes candida en masse, and removes the toxicity that the fungus calls home. It also creates an alkaline, oxygen-rich, internal environment—which is an environment where candida, cancer, and many other pathogens have a hard time living and often can't exist. In any case, you'll see the candida and filth come out of you each and every day, so you won't have any questions about the program's effectiveness. Many overgrowth situations can be eliminated in a few months by following these protocols and if you know anything about candida overgrowth, you'll understand that this is a minor miracle. More serious overgrowths, however, can take longer.

If you suffer from candida overgrowth, it's important that you do get rid of it, for your own sake and for the sake of everyone around you. When you understand that candida is implicated in depression, anger, mood swings, PMS, and other "emotional" disturbances, it's plain to see why eliminating your overgrowth will have positive effects on those around you. You might also want to look at the time, money, and energy you pour into health problems and consider how your resources could be better directed once your overgrowth is eliminated.

If you find cleansing difficult to sustain for extended periods of time, then do it for shorter periods and follow *The Cleaning Up! Diet* with lots of coconut oil between cleanses. (Ch. 7 & Appendix B) However, you'll want to cleanse regularly until your problem is at bay. The key is to keep at it until you've eliminated your overgrowth, or at least the large majority of it, because sometimes the nitty-gritty can be a bit tricky.

Test for Candida Overgrowth

Now, for the big question: Do you have candida overgrowth?

The spit test is a simple test that can indicate the presence of a candida overgrowth problem. In my years of working with candida issues, I've found this test has remarkable accuracy. You look at your spit because your tongue reflects what's going on in your entire body. So if you have the overgrowth anywhere in your body, it will be reflected in your tongue and therefore in your spit. If you test positive, candida cleansing can be one of the best things you've ever done for yourself.

The spit test:

First thing in the morning—before you brush your teeth or put anything into your mouth—gather the saliva in your mouth and spit into a clear glass filled with lukewarm tap water.

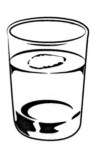

Now set the glass down and after about fifteen minutes, hold the glass about eye level and examine your spit. If your body is free of candida overgrowth, your spit will float at the top in a small clump or be around the sides of the glass, without any of the signs below. If you have candida overgrowth, you will likely see one or more of the following signs:

✳ Cloudy white matter which originates from the spit and "hangs" down toward the bottom of the glass

✳ A white sediment in the water or at the bottom of the glass

✳ Spit that is spread out across the top of the water with a "web-like" material holding it together.

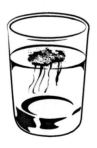 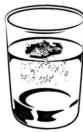 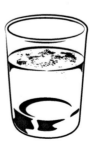

These are listed in order of severity (with the most severe first) and the more that occur, often indicates a more severe case of candida overgrowth. Depending on the extent of your initial situation, the length of your cleanse, and the degree and aggressiveness you follow these protocols, your spit will either clear up entirely or gradually improve.

You can also do this test to help determine when your situation has been eliminated. But know that this test is sensitive. If you have a little candida problem somewhere in your body—even a small clump that you're having a hard time reaching—it can show a problem, even if you've removed (and seen removed) a tremendous amount with this program.

Chapter 4

The ABCs of Cleansing: How and Why

Now let's talk about how this program works. I believe that knowledge is power, and especially when it comes to caring for your body, you'll need to know exactly what you're doing and why. So, let's take a closer look at the methods.

Diet Modification

On this program, you'll be feeding your body pure nutrition for optimal cleansing and you'll avoid feeding candida overgrowth. So, you'll be loading up on vegetables and avoiding sugars, carbohydrates, meat, and dairy. You'll also be taking in plenty of nutrition through fresh juices, particularly sweet green juices, that are mineral-rich and highly detoxifying. In addition, many of your meals will be raw—or uncooked— so they'll contain the enzymes necessary for your body to break them down, which eases the burden on your digestive system. Enzymes are powerful substances. They help break down foods, cleanse the body, and they also initiate every action in the body—including functions like blinking and breathing. Because of this, enzymes are often called our "life force" and literally when we run out of enzymes, we die.

Enzymes are present in all foods from nature, but they're destroyed by heat and processing, so if you're not eating plenty of raw foods from nature, you're draining your enzyme reserves and your life force. Eating foods from nature in their raw, uncooked state, also avoids adding to the body all of the different molecular combinations that are constantly created from heating foods—and gets us back as close as possible to a truly natural diet.

With this type of diet, most people will be dramatically decreasing their incoming toxic load, by substantially reducing the number of chemicals coming in from processed foods. Most people will also substantially *increase* their nutrients coming in, by eating heartily from nature's foods.

Another little-known fact is that the human body uses up to 30 percent of all of the energy it produces each day, simply to digest food. So, when you eat in ways that give your digestive system a break that "extra" energy goes toward cleaning and healing your body—something your body doesn't always have time for when it's busy digesting complicated foods. As this energy is redirected, your body will also start eliminating its most inferior tissue and cleaning out toxic matter from your organs, fat, and cells—which is an important part of the cleansing process. If you're up for it, you can intensify this by adding the fasting component in the "Super-charge Your Cleanse" chapter.

Colon Cleansing

In addition to diet modification, *The Cleaning Up! Cleanse* uses regular enemas to ensure you're eliminating all of the toxins released by the diet modification program— and to remove other waste that you've been unable to dispose of naturally. Unfortunately, the average person has ten or more pounds of *old*, rotten fecal matter in his or her colon—including a hardened, toxic, rubber-like substance known as mucoid plaque.

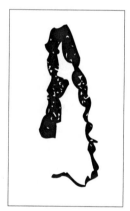

Mucoid Plaque

Why is this a problem? First, that's *a lot* of putrefying waste in the body. Second, an unclean colon leaks toxicity to nearby organs and feeds toxic matter to *every* cell in the body through the bloodstream. Of course, every cell in the body includes cells in the brain and nervous system— exacerbating problems for those prone to anger, nervousness, depression, and other emotional problems.

Mucoid plaque might be a new concept for you.[4] It's formed because your body produces mucus as a protective coating for your colon walls when you ingest substances that your

---

4   To learn more about mucoid plaque, read Dr. Richard Anderson's book, *Cleanse and Purify Thyself.*

body considers harmful. But, unfortunately, what the *body* considers harmful and what the average twenty-first century *mind* considers harmful are often two different things!

When all of the mucus isn't eliminated—which is common because it's sticky and our fiber intake is generally low, the mucus hardens—and mucoid plaque forms. If poor dietary habits were only occasional, then the mucus would be produced only in small amounts and our bodies would be able to eliminate it. However, in most people, the mucus is produced continually and never totally eliminated. It's left in the colon to harden into mucoid plaque—which is extraordinarily toxic.

For many, this process starts in childhood and when mucoid plaque builds in the colon, it generally stays put until some deep colon cleansing is done. You're likely to see mucoid plaque pass while on *The Cleaning Up! Cleanse*—many people pass several feet of it. So, watch for long strands or a ball of tar-like matter—and if you see these, be glad they're now on the outside, rather than still stuck on the inside!

A clean colon is an essential part of the cleansing process and it shouldn't be overlooked. But in this program, we use enemas for far more than just cleaning the colon...

Enemas to Clean the Liver

After some initial colon cleansing, *coffee enemas* are introduced to clean the liver. Your liver is arguably your body's most important organ and it's definitely your hardest working organ. Unlike other organs with just a handful of jobs, your liver has *more than a thousand jobs*—and two of its primary tasks are detoxification and burning fat.

Actually, your liver is so important that compromising its ability to detoxify daily is your fastest way to poor health. An overburdened liver also makes weight loss incredibly difficult, because your liver will prioritize detoxification over burning fat. This is why keeping your liver in top shape is the easiest way to lose weight and to maintain your ideal weight once you've achieved it.

Unfortunately, though, most people's livers are in a poor state. Also, unfortunately, liver tests from a doctor generally won't show a problem unless it's a life-threatening condition. But the fact is: most people's livers are largely storage sites for toxins that the liver couldn't render harmless. Your liver just does you the favor of *storing* the toxins—instead of allowing them float freely in your blood. But when this happens continuously, you simply reduce your liver's capacity to

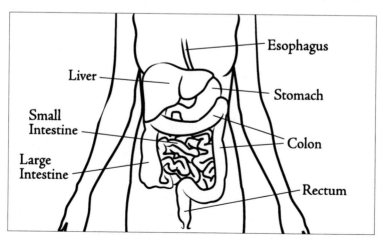

do its thousand other jobs—day in and day out—including daily detoxification and burning fat.

Coffee enemas have been used for nearly a century to detoxify the liver; they regularly help people regain their health, weight, and body's natural ability to detoxify itself. Coffee enemas have also been used *successfully* in cancer healing centers around the world for decades, attesting to how important the liver is in making or breaking health—and to how well these enemas work.

Enemas to Clean the Entire Body

The Cleaning Up! Cleanse then takes coffee enemas a step further and uses natural cleansing substances *with the coffee enemas* to reach in through the liver—and touch the bloodstream. Because all of the blood in the body travels through the liver every three minutes, these enemas allow us to simply and easily oxygenate the body to create an environment where many diseases and pathogens can't get a foothold. They also allow us to cleanse the body of candida, viruses, parasites, heavy metals, radiation and other chemical contamination—throughout the body.

All of the substances used with the coffee enemas are natural substances—they include baking soda, coconut oil, greens and other herbs and healing foods. This chapter and chapter 8 talk more about them. If these substances were taken by mouth, they would also end up in your liver and bloodstream. However, by inserting them directly into your liver with the coffee enemas, we can accomplish far more.

Of course, we induce this massive detoxification with enemas so the pathway *out of the body* is wide open—for quick and painless removal. Almost instantaneously, you can say goodbye to the candida and filth and rejoice at removing it for good. Most people will be amazed by what comes out, surprised at how much there is of it, and delighted that it's gone permanently!

The Massage Techniques

Remember those pockets of waste the body creates to contain and corral various poisons? The good news is: with self administered massage during the enemas with coffee and the other cleansing substances, we're often able to break up those pockets of waste and manually loosen the candida and filth contained within.

Using deep massage, you can break up the casing of the pockets and wring the toxicity out of them. You'll also be massaging your entire body to make waste contained *throughout your body* available for removal. The massage encourages blood flow to the areas you're massaging and brings the natural cleansing substances there—for them to do their amazing work. Your blood then brings the loosened filth to your liver, which immediately dumps the toxins into your colon for removal via the enemas. The removal of massive amounts of filth can be an almost instantaneous process.

It's also important to know that blood in the body flows like a river. So, blockages and stagnation upstream often mean pollution in that area *and downstream*. Knots and waste in the shoulders (seen as innocent tight shoulder muscles) can mean poor blood flow to the head and brain—which may manifest as allergies and problems with thinking, concentration, etc. It can also bring about more serious problems that affect the brain.

Toxicity in the lower back and hip areas can mean lack of blood flow to the lower extremities, and lead to back pain, bone misalignment, sore muscles, cold feet, etc. With pockets of waste blocking blood flow, your body is also restricted in its ability to deliver oxygen and cleanse itself properly—which can manifest all sorts of symptoms. Of course, waste near organs can affect the organ's ability to do its jobs—causing even more problems.

It's particularly exciting that with these special enemas and the massage techniques, we're for the first time able to target areas of the body to remove candida and general toxicity.

Build-up of Toxins Restricts Blood Flow

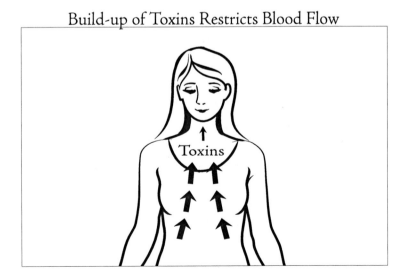

Toxins

This is critical because we can now target our areas of pain and disease to remove the toxicity at the root of the problem. After all, why live with it, when you can remove it?

The Supplements

The Cleaning Up! Cleanse uses several supplements to aid the cleansing process so, let's take a minute and talk about them and why they're used.

Psyllium husk powder is standard in many cleansing programs and is used for two reasons. First, psyllium is a very effective colon cleanser. It scrubs years of built-up filth from large and small intestines, and does a good job of dislodging mucoid plaque for removal. Second, because psyllium expands in your stomach, it helps keep you full—which is wonderful when you're changing your diet. If you ever feel hungry, just have more to eat or have a drink with psyllium to fill you up.

Virgin coconut oil is used because it's incredibly detoxifying and it's a powerful anti-fungal, anti-viral, anti-bacterial, and anti-parasitic agent.[5] It plays a key role in *The Cleaning Up! Cleanse* because coconut oil kills candida and many other pathogens quickly—and dramatically shortens the time required for deep and thorough cleansing.

Coconut oil is also a healthy fat that speeds up the metabolism (by as much as 60 percent!) and, believe it or not, helps

---

5   To learn more about the incredible powers of coconut oil, read *Coconut Cures* or *The Coconut Oil Miracle*—both by Bruce Fife.

overweight people lose weight. If, on the other hand, you have no weight to lose, coconut oil will help you maintain your weight. Coconut oil is known to improve thyroid func-

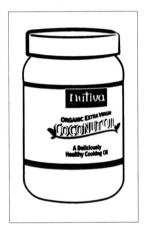

tion, protect the heart, and halt the growth of cancer cells. Because cancer grows in the body for *years* before it can be detected, this is important for just about everybody.

In *The Cleaning Up! Cleanse,* we use coconut oil orally (in many of the recipes), topically (as a lotion), and with the coffee enemas to get the maximum benefits from this miracle oil. Consuming coconut oil aids in eliminating candida overgrowth in the intestines and throughout the body. In the enemas, coconut oil produces powerful candida elimination results throughout the body and kills candida *en masse* in between enema sessions. Topical use of the oil has the same anti-fungal and anti-bacterial benefits—plus it's highly moisturizing and provides a natural sunscreen. Coconut oil's anti-viral, anti-bacterial, and weight loss or maintenance properties make it helpful even for those who don't have candida problems.

Coconut oil once had an undeserved reputation for being an unhealthy saturated fat. That was before researchers understood that there are two types of saturated fats: long chain and medium chain. Saturated fats from animals are long chain—and are truly bad for you. However, coconut oil is different. Coconut oil is a medium chain fatty acid—which has tremendous health benefits. Medium chain fatty acids are found only a few places in nature and another one is in mother's milk. In breast milk, these germ-fighting fatty acids *protect* the infant as the immune system develops. This is one of the reasons breast-fed infants regularly have better health than formula-fed infants.

Baking soda is another key supplement and it's a naturally occurring alkaline mineral. Baking soda
is common in baking and club
soda—and it also can be used to
create an alkaline environment in
the body. Alkaline is the term used
when the body has more *oxygen*
than hydrogen (which is acidic).
It's important for the body to be
oxygen-rich and slightly alkaline,
because candida, cancer, parasites, harmful bacteria, and many other pathogens *struggle to survive* in oxygen-rich alkaline environments—whereas these problems *thrive* in acidic oxygen-deprived environments.[6]

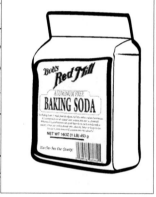

So, remember acids and bases from your high school chemistry class? Bases neutralize acids. In this case, baking soda is the base we'll use to neutralize acidic toxins in your body. Using baking soda is an easy way to neutralize toxins and

6   To learn more about the importance of being slightly alkaline and that many health problems stem from being acidic, check out *The pH Miracle* by Robert O. Young, PhD.

internal stores of filth because *all toxins and filth are acidic* — and it takes twenty times as much base to neutralize an acid.

Interestingly, the medical community uses baking soda—also called sodium bicarbonate—intravenously when a condition called metabolic acidosis occurs. Metabolic acidosis is the term for a body with excessive stored acids.

Believe it or not, sodium bicarbonate is natural in the body too. In fact, your body naturally produces sodium bicarbonate to create a buffer against common metabolic acids. The problem is: we don't create enough for our highly acidic twenty-first-century lifestyles. Well, actually the problem is our highly acidic twenty-first century lifestyles—and using baking soda is a way to correct the problems they've created.

To understand why the average person is so acidic, you need to know that what you eat has a huge effect on whether you're acidic or alkaline. With the exception of most raw fruits and vegetables, most foods are acidic. The worst offenders are meat, dairy, processed foods, and sugary foods. In addition, stress, pollution, negative thinking, and common chemicals all create an acidic internal environment. With this knowledge, it's easy to see why most of us have been acidic for years!

Using baking soda creates a rush of oxygen in the body and an environment where the offending pathogens disintegrate and often become available for removal. The stored toxins react with the baking soda, resulting in the neutralization of the acid and the formation of carbon dioxide (which is excreted through the lungs) and water. Actually, the acidic hydrogen becomes one of the H2s in the water in your urine or removed with the enemas. Essentially, the harmful waste in your body is turned into harmless compounds, which are immediately removed. Of course, this aids tremendously in detoxification and is extraordinarily helpful in loosening the pockets of waste we've discussed so they can be removed.

Many find it interesting to know that an oncologist in Rome, Dr. Tullio Simoncini, has been eliminating cancers by injecting a baking soda solution directly into them. The cancers regularly disappear and sometimes in a matter of days![7] Dr. Simoncini's work is fascinating and he clearly states that cancer is an advanced form of candida overgrowth. Personally, I think Dr. Simoncini is onto something *and* that there's more to it.

Many of the solid lumps or "pockets of waste" I broke down in my own body contained "balls" of candida. The lumps were also often held together by candida and another, harder, casing. In addition to having balls of candida, the lumps were filled with *large amounts of filth.* I actually believe that cancers and tumors are part of the body's way of *containing* the chemicals, heavy metals, viruses and filth that the body doesn't have the resources to eliminate—and this would explain why so many chemicals and pathogens *cause* cancer. But, with time and accumulation, the containment site simply becomes a problem.

In any case, in this program, you'll use baking soda in a drink with psyllium husk powder and you'll use it in the enemas.

---

7   You can learn more from Dr. Simoncini's book, *Cancer is a Fungus.*

It's also used in the coffee enemas to bring the remarkable benefits of baking soda throughout your body to dislodge and remove enormous amounts of filth.

You should know that many holistic health practitioners recommend drinking baking soda for digestive issues, and Dr. Simoncini recommends drinking it for cancers of the intestinal track. You should also know that baking soda has a pH of 8, which is just slightly more alkaline than where our blood is meant to be, which is pH 7.34 (7 is neutral while above 7 is alkaline and below 7 is acidic.) However, compare that to the other end of spectrum of what people commonly do. Soft drinks, for example, are often in the pH range of 2.3 to 4—being highly acidic, and *much* further away from where our blood pH is meant to be. Yet, a great deal of our society doesn't think twice about drinking them. Baking soda is also known to dissolve and prevent many kidney stones.

Probiotics are healthy bacteria for our colon and the ideal colon balance is 80 percent "good" bacteria and 20 percent

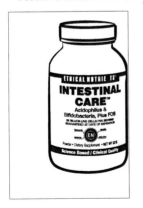

"bad" bacteria. Yet, most people have the portions reversed! People with candida issues should know the very fact that they have candida attests to an unhealthy balance of bacteria in their colon. Folks with IBS should heed the same warning.

Everyone, however, should *always* replenish his or her healthy bacteria after colon cleansing. So, in *The Cleaning Up! Cleanse*, we use probiotic supplements and raw sauerkraut to replenish and rebuild these important bacteria in our bodies. While probiotic supplements contain more concentrated healthy bacteria, sauerkraut is important too, because it can contains *more and different strains* of healthy bacteria.

Chapter 5

How You Might Feel

You may feel absolutely wonderful on this program, and after you've released a significant amount of toxicity, you'll probably feel better than you have in years. But let's face it: with any type of deep cleaning, sometimes it gets worse before it gets better.

Detox Symptoms

Because you'll be releasing many toxins and they'll need to come out of their hiding places before they can be removed, at times you may experience detoxification symptoms. Detoxification symptoms are just symptoms the body exhibits with high levels of toxins in the blood and common ones include headaches, acne, fevers, bad breath, body odor, sore muscles, feelings of nausea, unusual tiredness, "spaciness," lack of coordination, poor moods, and cold- or flu-like symptoms. You may also relive a past illness, and feel it again briefly, as the source of the problem has been dislodged and is exiting your body. People sometimes also feel the effects of long ago taken pharmaceuticals, as they are finally being removed from the body.

So, if any of this happens, it's important to understand what's happening and why it's happening. Because if you don't understand how detoxification can work, you'll think you're getting sick, when you're actually getting healthy. If you're experiencing detoxification symptoms, just let your body do its thing, and make sure to use the methods in the "Minimizing Detox Symptoms" chapter to speed the process. You can eliminate many detoxification symptoms immediately with an enema (by getting those now loosened toxins out of your body). But also know that having some detoxification symptoms is a normal part of the cleansing process, and unless they're extreme, they're nothing to be concerned about. And if they're extreme, it's a sign that you should at least slow your cleanse.

If you believe the enemas or colonics (if you're doing them) caused your detox symptoms, it's actually a sign that you need more. You've just loosened some waste in your colon and haven't gotten it out fast enough for your body's liking.

If you aren't feeling well or develop flu-like symptoms, the absolute worst thing you can do is take medication. Drug methods generally suppress our natural elimination methods and inadvertently store our toxins *in* our bodies, which only serves to create more problems down the road. Actually, the suppression of our natural detoxification methods is the reason some drugs appear to work, but because they don't address the root cause of toxicity, people choosing this route will often experience more problems, and more serious problems, down the road.

So, understand that detoxification symptoms can be part of the cleansing process and simply how people feel with too many toxins in their bloodstream. In fact, when you understand how the body behaves with too many toxins in the bloodstream, it may change the way you view illness—because many common "illnesses" are just signs of toxicity and the body's attempt to remove or contain those toxins.

For example, fevers heat the body so that toxins can be eliminated through the skin. Vomiting removes toxins en masse from the stomach. Diarrhea does the same from the bowel. Sneezing removes toxins from the sinuses, and coughing is a way to clean the lungs. Acne and rashes are just toxins coming out through the skin. I also believe that cancers, tumors, and other lumps are part of the body's way of clumping together toxins with candida—to keep them out of the bloodstream.

It's really to our benefit to understand what's going on when we experience any of these things and *help our bodies eliminate the toxins they need to eliminate*, instead of using drug methods to stop the detoxification process, and store the toxins inside of us.

In any case, whether you feel good or bad while cleansing depends entirely on where you are in regards to toxin removal. Discomfort is often followed by clarity when the toxins are released. So, when toxins are heavy in your bloodstream and you feel discomfort, simply guide them out and you'll feel better soon.

Emotional Detoxification

On this program, you may detoxify emotionally, too. This is because your body sometimes stores toxic emotions from your past. Actually, I believe that stored negative emotions can be the energetic "glue" that binds toxins to certain areas in the body. Then, those stuck emotions can cause emotional blocks in us and subconsciously influence our behavior, often in negative ways. But who ever thinks these things are related to toxicity or that they could be removed with cleansing? However, when you remove the toxicity that binds the emotions in your body, the stored emotions are then free to leave your body.

The good news about this: when those negative emotions are no longer vibrating in your body, you'll be much less likely to feel them, or be triggered by them, in the future. And since subconscious stored negative emotions can be very destructive in people's lives, the effects can be almost miraculous when they're experienced.

Stored toxic emotions can run the gamut from fear, sadness, worry, nervousness, or anger. They can also be related to a specific instance in your past, of which you may become aware of as you're releasing it. In any case, when detoxifying emotionally, you may briefly feel these emotions as they leave your body and you'll definitely need to understand what's going on. If you're feeling offending emotions, an enema is usually the fastest way to move them out of your body and more techniques to clear negative energy are in Chapter 12.

You'll also be happy to know that not all physical or emotional detoxification is accompanied by feeling badly, in fact *most of the time, it isn't*. But since it *can* happen, it's important that you understand what's going on, why it's happening, and what to do about it.

Cleansing Can Feel Wonderful, Too!

Now let's talk about the good stuff that comes with cleansing, because there really is far more good than bad. Feelings of euphoria, extreme mental clarity, clearer vision, spiritual awakening, elevated thought, peace, and steadiness of nerves are common experiences when cleansing—and can become pretty much standard once you have a clean body. *Isn't it amazing that we can create this?*

These experiences are common after large amounts of toxins have been released—because a clean body no longer struggles to overcome its toxic burden and energy can flow freely throughout the body, as toxic blocks are removed. Actually, I believe these elevated consciousnesses are our *natural states of consciousness*—and it's only our toxic burden that regularly pulls us into lower emotional consciousnesses.

Interestingly, though, I'm far from the first to speak of the connection between our higher power and the state of our body—which is directly influenced by what we put into it. It's plain as day in the story of Adam and Eve, whose fall from grace (disconnection from our divine source) was, literally interpreted, caused by *eating foods they weren't supposed to be eating*.

In fact, the story of Adam and Eve may be the story of humankind's fall from spiritual connectedness when humans started *cooking their foods*. To understand how this possibly could have taken place, you have to understand that when we cook foods, we change their molecular structure. And by making changes to a diet entirely from nature, we change the degree of toxicity we'll have, whether we're acidic or alkaline, literally what molecules are in our system, and as a consequence, how we'll function. When you change the input, there will be changes in the output.

The loss of our easily obtained spiritual connection may be just one the effects that regularly occurs from non-natural diets—including ones as normal to us as cooked foods—followed by others like health, weight and emotional problems. If you think about it, the story tells us they fell from eating foods from the center of the garden. Well, at the time the whole Earth was a garden, and *fire* is what's at the center of the Earth. So, it's very possible that this story is telling us that they "fell," or became disconnected, from eating fired, or cooked, foods.

They also fell, according to the story, from eating from the tree of knowledge of good and evil. It's possibly this occurred because: Before humans started cooking their food, *they knew no evil*. In truth, there aren't even hints of organized war before humans started cooking their foods a few hundred thousand years ago. Researchers have also found, by accident at first, that rats will tolerate each other in tight quarters on a pure, raw food diet. But, one rat often kills the other in the same quarters, less than 24 hours after eating cooked bread or cheese[8]. With an understanding of how fundamentally common foods can affect emotions and therefore behavior, one has to wonder how much violence, fear, and aggression in our society is really caused by humans regularly eating improper diets, and their toxic effects.

This interpretation also connects perfectly with the enhanced spiritual connections that many people who have deeply cleansed and follow pure raw food diets enjoy. And seriously, have you ever noticed that the devil is regularly portrayed with *fire and a fork*? There's really a lot more to food, the state of our bodies, and spirituality than most people realize.

So, in a time when pesticides, genetically altered foods, processed foods, thousands of chemicals *and* cooked foods are common everyday faire, this might be something you want to consider carefully. Although you might be more likely to believe it really could be a truthful interpretation once you've cleansed deeply and are enjoying a pure raw food diet—and are experiencing the differences for yourself.

Actually, it's not coincidental that historical individuals known for their spirituality, including Jesus, Buddha, and St. Francis of Assisi—all cleansed deeply through extensive fasting before beginning their teachings. It appears that even in far less toxic times, these men needed *to detoxify* in order to enhance and perhaps obtain, their connection to our divine source.

---

8   For more on this and hoe we only became a war-based society *after* we started altering our natural diets, read *GeneFit Nutrition* by Roman Devivo and Antje Spors.

In *The Gospel of Peace,* Jesus even gave enema instructions and said "the uncleanness within is far greater than the uncleanness without." It turns out that Jesus was deeply into cleansing and conscious eating—and he connected it with our spirituality too.

In any case, by eating foods of inferior quality and failing to remove the problems of the past through deep cleansing, I believe we make the direct connection to our divine source difficult or impossible on an energetic level. I think it's likely due to our acidic state, so much toxic inference, and a lack of life force energy from raw foods. Yet, if we deviate too far energetically, we often lose our ability to obtain and maintain the connection. And unfortunately, if we lose this connection, it's all too easy to connect with lower energy sources, which are fear-based and the source of anger, fear, worry, judgment, and other energetically negative emotions, which influence our behavior. Of course, our behavior can cause us to disconnect too, but as we've already talked about, our emotions and subsequently our behavior can be influenced—in ways we're largely unconscious of—through our diets and stored toxicity.

I bring this up because if our common foods, our toxic, acidic bodies, and our chemical-based lifestyles really *are* how the human race regularly disconnects from our divine source and therefore is the hidden root of so many of the negative things we see in our world, I think at a minimum, we should know about it. I also think that understanding the cause of the problem is the only way to work backward to reverse it, and then prevent it from continuing.

Chapter 6

Minimizing Detox Symptoms

Since detoxification symptoms are a reflection of the mobilization of stored toxins, the way to minimize them is to move those toxins out of your body *as quickly as possible*. These methods will help you do just that and the first two are good protocols whenever you're not feeling well—cleansing or not. Remember: many common "illnesses" are just your body's way of removing harmful substances, so the more you expedite the process, the better off you'll be.

Sometimes people also get a bit scared if their detoxification symptoms are extreme, so it's important to remember that detoxification symptoms only happen if you're feeling your own stored toxins. And from a larger picture perspective, the problem is really that these toxins are in your body—not any reactions you might have as they are being removed. Sometimes people also want to cut back on the enemas, and if you've been cleansing a while, or you've done a lot of deep cleansing before coming to this program, that's absolutely fine. However, this program offers a deep and aggressive cleanse, and especially in the beginning, most people will feel much better if they are doing the enemas more aggressively, rather than less.

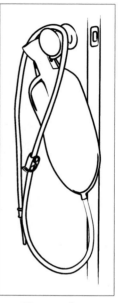

Enema bag

The Methods

1. Colon Cleansing

Colon cleansing releases a huge amount of toxins every time it's done, and it's one of the best ways to dump toxins quickly. So, if you're experiencing any detoxification symptoms, take a water enema, followed by a coffee enema. This generally does the trick pretty quickly by speeding those toxins out of your body. The only thing you can do wrong here is to fail to clean your colon and liver regularly while you cleanse. If you're experiencing detoxification symptoms, and it's at all possible, it's also best to do these enemas twice a day until they've passed.

2. Lots of Water

Extra water supports your kidneys and sweeps those toxins out of your body. Herbal teas and fresh juices are great too, however for detoxification symptoms, I'd pass on the green drinks as they will initiate deeper detoxification.

3. Slow Your Cleanse

If you're feeling awful and these methods aren't helping, you're likely detoxifying too rapidly. In which case, it's best to slow your cleanse. To slow your cleanse temporarily eliminate the coconut oil and start eating the cooked vegetable meals. You can also skip the baking soda and psyllium drinks and if you're doing any of the Super-charge methods (Chapter 12), just hold off until you're feeling better.

Actually, if you think you might be on the more toxic side, ie, lots of pharmaceuticals, current or past heavy cigarette use, a serious disease or many illnesses, a mostly processed or fast food diet, etc., you can also *start* your cleanse in this manner, and add the rest in a week or two into the process.

Other Things You Might Experience

A Little Colder—A large portion of your body heat is generated from digestion, so especially if you're cleansing in cooler weather, you might need to bundle up a bit and drink warm teas. It's also not uncommon for the hands and feet to become colder, so wearing extra socks is a good idea too.

Light-headed - You can feel a little light-headed when cleansing, and you may experience visual darkness if you stand up quickly. Stand up slowly to prevent this and know that if it does, it's harmless.

Water Retention—Baking soda can cause water retention and the best way to alleviate this is to have a half cup of parsley each day in a fresh-squeezed or blended juice.

The Hiccups—People sometimes get the hiccups after consuming baking soda in the drinks, but generally this goes away as your body becomes accustomed to it.

Tingling in Your Body—During cleansing with the baking soda, you may occasionally feel a tingling in your body, perhaps in your feet or limbs. This is just oxygenated blood reaching the area—and it's a good thing. Generally, it doesn't last long.

A Coated Tongue—These are toxins your body is releasing and the same toxin-dumping process is going on throughout your entire body. As you become cleaner internally, so will your tongue.

A Little Tired—While cleansing, you may feel a little tired, for a few reasons. You may have dislodged some waste, and you'll be tired until you've removed it with an enema. Or, if you're using the baking soda aggressively, it can be draining due to its oxygenating effects. In addition, cleansing can be taxing on the body over an extended period.

The green drinks and liver tonics are helpful in boosting energy when cleansing (Appendix C) and be sure to take breaks from the enemas if you need them. Also know— without a doubt—you're going to be far better off with all of your stored waste *outside* your body, even if you are a little tired during the process. However, if you're extremely tired over an extended period, it's best to end your cleanse for a while or take more breaks from the enemas. You can always come back to cleansing, but you're drained, it's better to take some time off until you've regained your strength.

Chapter 7

Preparing Delicious Meals

The Cleaning Up! Cleanse entails switching to a primarily vegetable diet which includes hearty salads, raw soups, homemade dressings, raw vegetable wraps, steamed vegetables, vegetable sautés, raw sauerkraut, and fresh juices with lots of sweet green drinks. Carbohydrates and most fruit are avoided as both feed candida and make it grow. However, for those without candida issues or sugar sensitivities, it's fine to include a variety of fresh fruit.

Since coconut oil is so beneficial in cleansing and candida killing, you'll be consuming quite a bit of it. Coconut oil will be your primary cooking oil, and it's used liberally in the soups and dressings.

Of course, you'll need delicious meals that are easy to prepare—and there are tons of easy, delicious vegetable meals for you to indulge in. Appendices B and C are packed full of them. But, be sure not to get these recipes confused with the ones in Appendix E, as those are to help you upgrade your ongoing diet after you're candida-free.

The raw vegetable meals are far more cleansing than the other options, so you should eat plenty of these meals—especially the salads and coconut oil soups. In fact, the salads, coconut oil soups, and green drinks should make up the bulk of your diet. Then, just add a cup or two of sauerkraut each week, and have whatever else in the diet you enjoy to meet your hunger, taste, and nutrition needs.

If you're short on time to prepare foods, the blended juices (as opposed to the juiced juices) are much faster to make, and the clean up only entails rinsing out your blender. And remember: your meals, especially your salads, should be large to make sure you're taking in plenty of nutrition and to avoid hunger. Your salads might be two or three times bigger than salads you're used to making—so, use the recipes (Appendix B), they're very different from standard mostly-lettuce salads.

To make your transition easier, might also want to enjoy some of these meals before beginning to cleanse. For many, it helps to experience how easy these meals are to prepare and how good they taste.

Because getting rid of major toxicity and candida problems can take some time, this cleanse also allows for a few foods that aren't ideal for candida cleansing to help you stick to the diet, if they're needed. However, if you're cleansing short-term (under two months), try and avoid the foods in the "In Small Amounts, If at All" section. Now let's look at which foods are candida-safe, which are not, and address a couple of common questions.

Candida-safe Foods for Cleansing

✳ Vegetables: asparagus, spinach, carrots, cabbage, green beans, peas, radishes, onions, broccoli, lettuce, celery, eggplant, leeks, bok choy, fennel, cilantro, parsley, cucumber, kale, any greens, sea vegetables, mushrooms, artichokes, brussels sprouts, peppers, ginger, garlic and other herbs.

✳ *Organic* zucchini and yellow crookneck squash can be eaten if they're peeled, as they often attract a mold while growing. Sprouts can also be eaten, but if you sprout them yourself, use caution, as it's easy for them to develop a little mold while sprouting. Store-bought sprouts are actually preferred.

✳ Essentially, all vegetables *except* potatoes, sweet potatoes, yams, corn, juiced carrots, beets* and tray grown wheatgrass. Tray grown wheatgrass is often contaminated with a mold growing on the bottom, however if you can lift up the tray and confirm that there isn't mold on the bottom, it should be fine.

✳ Fruit: tomato, avocado, lemon, lime, grapefruit, green apples and berries. Grapefruit, green apples and berries and should be used as whole fruit (not juiced) and used sparingly. Grapefruit and berries can be sweetened with stevia. (If you're having a sweet craving, try countering it with a green apple blended with blueberries, a little water, and stevia.)

---

*   Beets can be used later in the program, See Chapter 12 for more.

* Seasonings: Sea salt, sesame oil, organic miso, organic naturally brewed shoyu, organic naturally brewed tamari
* Sweetener: Stevia, a sugar-free herbal sweetener
* Herbal teas: all except those with chamomile
* Oils: Virgin coconut oil, cold-pressed olive oil, sesame oil
* Store bought raw, unpasteurized sauerkraut.
* Some foods like raw kale, spinach, parsley, broccoli, cabbage, asparagus, cilantro, garlic, onion, and beets* do double duty for cleansing, often killing pathogens or boosting our own detoxification enzymes. The more of these you can enjoy in your meals and juices, the better.

In Small Amounts, If at All

* Nuts and seeds are generally healthy, but many of them are contaminated with an invisible mold, which has a detrimental effect on candida. However, if you're going to be cleansing for a length of time (over a few months), eating nuts and seeds can help you maintain your strength and keep weight on, if it's needed. So, if needed or desired, add a cup or two of raw, soaked nuts or seeds to your diet each week. Just soak them in probiotic water as described in Appendix E which can help remove some of the mold. Nuts and seeds can be eaten raw or blended into several soups and salad dressings. (Appendix B) Almonds, macadamia, and pistachios shouldn't be used as they're often contami-

nated. Peanuts also shouldn't be consumed. Sunflower seeds, brazil nuts, cashews, and pumpkin seeds are best as they're less often contaminated.

✶ While avoiding the sugar in fruit is important for candida problems, if you're having a hard time with the diet because of sweet or other cravings, a little fresh fruit might be just what's needed to make it doable.

✶ Beans and lentils can have a slightly negative effect on candida, but if you're regularly hungry they can provide the substance you may need for long-term cleansing. (Recipes, Appendix E)

Candida-feeding Foods to Avoid

Everything you eat plays a role in determining the fate of candida problems and a number of substances, including sugar and carbohydrates, feed candida and make it grow, undermining your efforts to eliminate it. Here's a list of foods that feed candida and when you eat any of them, you take a step backward with candida and, except the fruit or vegetable juices, general cleansing too. You'll need to know this list well, and if you eat pre-prepared or restaurant foods check to make sure none of these ingredients are in the mix.

✶ Sugar in all forms (read labels carefully for sucrose, fructose, maltose, cane sugar, brown sugar, high-fructose corn syrup, corn syrup)

✶ Carbohydrates in general: grains, cereals, bread, potatoes, rice, pasta, popcorn, tortillas, crackers, etc.

✶ Products containing wheat, flour or yeast

✱ Alcohol, especially beer and wine

✱ Fruit juices and sweet vegetable juices including beet and carrot

✱ Non-organic animal products, as they contain hormones, antibiotics and likely genetically modified genes

✱ All dairy, except occasional organic butter and unsweetened organic yogurt

✱ Vinegar and foods with vinegar in it (read the labels)

✱ Otherwise healthful sweeteners, including maple syrup, honey, and agave

✱ Sodas, junk food and coffee

✱ Processed or smoked animal products

✱ Any food with mold on it, including blue cheese. Choose your veggies and berries carefully and use caution with leftovers. Cauliflower regularly has a visible black mold and recently I've been seeing raspberries with a visible fungus.

✱ Chamomile tea

It's not recommended, but if you must do alcohol while cleansing long term, your best option is vodka with soda water (not tonic water, as tonic water contains sugar). It's good with the juice of half a lemon or lime, and if you add a little stevia, it's fabulous. Of course, vodka is recommended only in small amounts. Wine and beer are both made with yeast, which will aggravate candida.

Simple Recipes

All of the recipes are extremely simple and based on simple concepts. So, have a look; they're a far cry from most recipes, which many people can find intimidating. Actually, the only real skill needed for most of the meals is chopping the veggies and from there it's often a simple blend or sauté away. Most of the meals also take ten minutes or less to prepare.

Protein Needs

If you are concerned about your protein needs, you should know that most estimates are that protein should be 10 to 15 percent of your diet, and most vegetables are 20 percent protein. So even on veggies alone, you'll be getting plenty of protein! However, when considering your protein needs, you should also know that most people have spent their lives taking in too much protein through animal consumption and for a few months, giving your body a chance to eliminate some of that excess protein will be beneficial.

However, if you're not convinced, you can get additional protein from nuts, seeds, beans, lentils, or a Spirulina supplement. Mushrooms and seaweed are also excellent protein options. Seaweed, specifically nori, is a great source of B-12 too.

Eating While Working

The lettuce-free salads (Appendix B) are simple to make and are easily incorporated in a working schedule. You can prepare them in the morning or take a bag of veggies to the office and cut them up there. The salad dressings can also be prepared a day in advance and transported in their own container. But, if you use avocado in a pre-prepared salad or dressing, squeeze lemon or lime over it to keep it fresh.

If you can, bring a blender to work too. It's great to have on hand to make extra blended green juices, soups, or dressings—whenever you like. Just rinse it when you're done and bring it home occasionally for a more thorough cleaning. You can also make your juices in the morning and bring them with you, ideally keeping them refrigerated and away from light.

Eating in Restaurants

Often you'll need to ask restaurants for special preparations and an easy way to enjoy restaurant meals is to simply prepare one of the salad dressings, bring it with you, and then order a large salad as your meal. Many times though, you'll need to ask them to leave off certain ingredients and you can also ask your server to add to your salad any candida-approved foods that you see elsewhere on the menu.

Many restaurants also offer steamed vegetables as a side dish and often times, you can have them prepare a large plate as a whole meal. If you have any of the salad dressings with you, they can be a delicious topping. Or you can just do a simple lemon, sea salt and olive oil dressing.

Keeping Weight On

It's important to know that with cleansing your body will generally find a happy weight—which is often thin, but not too thin. And from that point, you generally won't lose any-more weight. However, if keeping weight on is important, just have more avocados, nuts, seeds, coconut oil, and beans or lentils, if you're including cooked foods. Using wild grass-es, which are discussed more in Appendix C, can help you keep muscle on while dissolving excess fat. All of these foods can help you feel full too, if you're feeling hungry.

Controversial Foods

If you know a lot about candida diets, you probably know that there are a few foods that even the experts can't seem to agree on. So, let's talk about a few, and I'll let you know my thoughts.

Fermented foods, like sauerkraut, are controversial with candida elimination, so here's the scoop. Generally speak-ing, vegetable-based fermented foods like sauerkraut are wonderful for cleansing and candida elimination because they are chock full of enzymes and healthy bacteria—and remember, it's the elimination of our healthy bacteria that often causes candida problems in the first place. However, occasionally fermented foods can become contaminated with unhealthy bacteria which is when they can be a problem—and if this happens they can feed problems like candida overgrowth. So, to avoid contamination issues but still benefit from fermented foods while cleansing, I recommend using only store bought *raw, unpasteurized* sauerkraut, which often is only found at health food stores.

Mushrooms also tend to be a bit controversial with candida. Because they're a fungus it's often thought that they feed fungal problems like candida overgrowth; it's a logic I once bought into myself. However, it turns out that many mushrooms are actually anti-fungal, powerful detoxifiers and allies in eliminating candida problems. Mushrooms are also great sources of protein and they're some of nature's most medicinal foods. It's interesting because the DNA of a mushroom is actually more similar to human DNA than to plant DNA, and the more I get into even common mushrooms, the more I believe that they're key foods that should be eaten raw and regularly for optimal health and vitality, especially for spiritual connectedness.

Mushrooms are the detoxifiers of the earth and due to the fact that many of them help with so many human diseases, part of me thinks they also do the same thing in our bodies. Mushrooms also spring from an underground communication network that to me is reminiscent of the spiritual connection that many of you will start experiencing, or begin experiencing more deeply, once you've done some deep cleansing and are eating mostly nature's raw foods. Personally, I think that regularly eating a variety of raw mushrooms is a way, in addition to cleansing, chemical avoidance, and raw foods, to develop this spiritual connectedness capacity in ourselves. Interestingly, it's even thought that mushrooms were the manna, or the bread of life, in the *Bible*.

Scholars that have studied the Dead Sea Scrolls have even come out saying that the early Christian movement, or what was actually taught and practiced by Christ and his disciples, revolved around mushrooms. You can Google it for more, but if you look, you'll start seeing mushrooms everywhere in early Christian art, and the art of other groups of spiritually connected people too. Some scholars think it's the psychedelic kind, but I noticed a big leap in myself when I started eating lots of raw portobello, shiitake, maitake, and crimini mushrooms—from a grocery store.

It gets interesting because I'm fairly sensitive, likely due my diet and the amount of cleansing I've done, and I can actually feel the back lower part of my brain start to activate after eating raw mushroom meals. And it turns out that this back lower portion of the brain is our love center. I can also feel it light up, if you will, when I am consciously manifesting things.

So, to make a long story short, I believe that eating plenty of raw mushrooms regularly helps us rewire or rebuild the love centers in our brains, which helps us develop our capacity for love-based living and probably also for manifesting that which is manifested in the consciousness of love. How's it done? I have no idea. In my mind, I always go back to the similar to human DNA and think mushrooms may play a role in bringing our DNA up a few notches, especially in this capacity. It's a theory, I know. But it's also well known that humans only use ten percent of their brains, and if you pick up any newspaper, you'll see we're not exactly the most loving of cultures.

Actually, taking it a step deeper, this would make mushrooms the body of Christ (some Biblical scholars would agree with this), and green drinks, or chlorophyll, the blood of Christ. Chlorophyll is well known to rebuild our blood and even create fresh blood.

Apple cider vinegar is another controversial of food in eliminating candida problems, and in truth, it's bit of a tricky one. On one hand, it does kill candida and on the other hand, it can become contaminated and feed it. And finally, it's working in the opposite direction of the alkaline environment we're working towards creating. For this reason, I recommend avoiding apple cider vinegar while cleansing for candida.

However, it's also not the worst thing you can do if you include a little in your diet, and personally, I think it makes great salad dressings. So, if you decide to use apple cider vinegar, I'd use it only occasionally in the salad dressings in Appendix E. It's also important that your apple cider vinegar is raw and unpasteurized.

All that said, if you're having problems with any of the foods in this section, or nuts or seeds, you can and should leave them out of your program.

Avoiding Genetically Altered Foods

Today we have something to look out for that no previous generation has ever had to pay attention to—genetically modified foods. GMO foods line most grocery store shelves even though they cause organ damage, especially reproductive damage, in animals—and sometimes death too.

Yet, in spite of the dangers, most people unknowingly eat genetically altered foods regularly. Of course, I recommend avoiding these foods *entirely* and since they're often not labeled, you'll need to know which foods are regularly genetically altered and avoid them with conscious buying habits.

The largest genetically altered crops are soy, corn, canola, sugar beets (which become white sugar), and cotton (which becomes apparel). As a rule, you shouldn't eat *any* of these foods if they're not organic, and avoid non-organic products made from them too. Common foods that are more than likely genetically altered if they're not organic are corn chips, corn oil, high fructose corn syrup, corn tortillas, tofu, miso, soy sauce, soybean oil, canola oil, cottonseed oil, margarine, tamari, shoyu, and white sugar. Many processed foods also contain canola oil, soy, corn, or white sugar, so avid label reading comes in handy. Some zucchini, yellow squash, and Hawaiian papaya are also genetically altered, and some flax has been contaminated too.

Animals are regularly fed genetically modified crops, and GM genes are in their meat and dairy too. Genetically modified genes have also been found to mix their genetic code with the healthy bacteria in humans *and* some GM genes are designed to produce pesticides continuously—so it's possible that many people now have gut bacteria that consistently produces its own pesticides.

Honestly, it's one of the most disturbing things I've come across in a while and if you want to know what I think the Biblical Mark of the Beast is, we're looking at it with the genetic manipulation of our own bodies from these scientifically derived "foods". Having the mark on the forehead means that people buy into GMOs mentally and on the right hand refers to the hand that most people eat with. It's also a bit difficult to buy and sell food without GMOs in them these days, unless you have a pure diet and are really paying attention.

In any case, in this cleanse, a few items from the list above are eaten, including shoyu (a fermented soy sauce), and these foods should *always* be organic. Of course, it's best to buy all of your foods organic, but when GMOs are involved, it's critical. Restaurants often use canola oil too, so if you're eating in restaurants, you'll need to check their oils. If it's a vegetable oil blend, it probably has genetically altered oils in the mix and it's best to pass on it, while also asking the restaurant to upgrade their oils. A complete non-GMO shopping guide can be found at www.nongmoshoppingguide. com/download.html and you'll also want to stay tuned to learn if other GMO foods are entering the market too.

Chapter 8

Colon Cleansing— Cleaning Up from the Inside Out!

As we've talked about, colon cleansing is critical to deep cleansing. Stored waste in the colon easily leaks throughout the body, and since the average person carries ten or more pounds of old fecal matter in his or her colon, it's important to get that filth out.

When you start colon cleansing, you will be amazed at what comes out of your own body. You will see, and unfortunately sometimes smell, some foul toxic waste that has probably been stored in your body for many years. It's putrid, it's rotten, and it's the cause of a significant number of diseases prevalent today. We're just not designed to have this filth sitting inside of us constantly.

The most effective and cost-effective way to correct this situation is with at-home enemas. Professional colonics are wonderful, yet while water colonics will effectively clean the filth from your large intestine, they won't allow for the deeper cleansing or massive candida elimination we're after in this program.

That said, it's a wonderful idea to start your cleansing with a series of professional colonics, if the cost is not prohibitive (about $75 each). Then you can transfer to at-home enemas to clean your liver, alkalize your body, and target candida, heavy metals, radiation, and other common problems.

If the cost of colonics is prohibitive, most people can do the initial cleansing just as effectively with at-home enemas. However, those with a larger gut, indicative of more impacted waste, would be wise to start with a series of four or more colonics in the first one to two weeks of their cleanse.

Some people are scared of enemas, but there is no reason to be. You really have more to fear from the filth that sits in your body if it's not cleaned out. Plus, enemas are simple, and not messy. All of the waste goes into the toilet, and nowhere else. And you're in the privacy of your own home with no one else around. So, have courage! *Try it.* Most people report that it's not anywhere near as bad as they had imagined. And take it from me—I used to be absolutely squeamish about enemas—they're not hard to do, uncomfortable, or even scary. Believe it or not, many people come to enjoy them!

Enema Ingredients

So, let's talk about the enema ingredients and what they do. Knowledge is power and this information is critical—if you want to live without major health, weight, and emotional problems.

Coffee

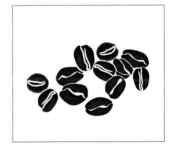

Coffee is used in enemas to remove large amounts of toxins from your liver. This is of the utmost importance because your liver is your main detoxification organ *and* your prime fat-burning organ. Yet, most people's liver's are overburdened by common lifestyles which mean that the body simply *can't* detoxify all of the chemicals ingested, inhaled, and applied to the body daily. An overburdened liver also doesn't prioritize burning fat—yet that's where many people are.

So, let's talk about coffee enemas and how they do this important job of detoxification. First, you'll need to know that your liver is under your right rib cage and it's connected to your colon by your bile ducts. Your bile ducts are the pathway your liver uses to dump the toxins it filters from your blood into your colon for removal. So, when the coffee solution fills your colon, it reaches your bile ducts. The solution then travels up your bile ducts and into your liver, and along the way the caffeine in the coffee expands, or dilates, your bile ducts. This temporarily opens the path from your liver to your colon and provides an open path for your liver to dump its stored toxins into your colon—which your liver does, happily and heartily. This massive dump of toxins is a blessing for our regularly overworked livers!

Since your liver filters all of your blood every three minutes, coffee enemas also clean your blood. They allow the toxins that your overburdened liver was previously unable to address to finally be filtered and dumped into your colon for removal. Of course, clean blood is foundational to good health.

For the majority of people, coffee in an enema will not have the same stimulating effect as coffee taken through the mouth, and even evening enemas should be fine. However, for a small percentage of individuals, coffee taken this way can have a caffeinating effect and if this is the case with you, reduce the amount of coffee used to one or two tablespoons and do your coffee-based enemas as early in the day as possible.

Baking Soda

As we've talked about, this program uses natural cleansing substances with coffee enemas, and baking soda is one of the substances used. Most people don't know it, but baking soda is actually a naturally occurring mineral found at the bottom of lakes. Of course, baking soda, or sodium bicarbonate, can also be manufactured, but naturally occurring baking soda is preferred on this program. Baking soda is a powerful enema ingredient because it quickly creates an alkaline oxygen-rich internal environment which is an environment where the bad guys disintegrate and become available for removal. Just as we can't survive without oxygen, many pathogens can't survive with it, so using baking soda is an easy way to remove a great deal of the harmful stuff from your body.

In this program, you'll use baking soda in a standalone enema to clean the candida and filth from your large intestine, and also as a pre-coffee enema to clean your colon before you introduce the coffee which will travel into your liver. Finally, you'll use baking soda combined with coffee enemas to bring the alkaline solution into your liver and therefore to your blood— for it to do its magic *throughout* your body.

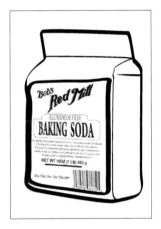

The coffee/baking soda enemas will quickly alkalize your body, immediately kill candida throughout your body, dislodge enormous amounts of filth, and aid in the removal of pockets of waste from your entire body. In addition, these enemas remove viruses and parasites from the body, and baking soda is known to absorb heavy metals and neutralize radiation too. And when you release, the filth will be immediately removed from your body.

Coffee Combination Enemas

In addition to baking soda, you can also add a number of herbs or foods with detoxification or medicinal qualities to your coffee or coffee and baking soda enemas. In truth, there are many foods and herbs from nature with healing properties that you can add for some amazing effects.

Greens are a standard on this cleanse, and you can also add any of the ones here to address specific problems and for desired results. Some of these might work better for some people than for others, so I recommend finding the ones that work best for you and using them regularly, while rotating them and trying new ones too. And the more filth you see coming out of you with each enema, the better. The more stars next to them, the more powerful I consider them to be. Mushroom and green enemas are also great for retention.

*****Wild grass - Amazing for overall detoxification. Especially great for cancer, lumps in the body, candida, fat burning, more energy, blood building, and diabetes. One of the most powerful detoxification enemas I've found; more about wild grasses at the end of this section and in Appendix C. (use one to three cups)

****Kale, parsley, spinach, chard, or other fresh greens - Powerful detoxifiers, great for candida, cancers, blood building, and lumps in the body. (use one to two cups)

****Maitake mushrooms - Great for cancer, lumps in the body, immune building, and detoxification. Great for diabetes, high blood pressure, and heart problems. With cancers, I'd make these a must. (use a ½ cup to a cup)

****Shiitake Mushrooms - Great for cancer, lumps in the body, and detoxification. A powerful anti-viral and immune booster; helps regulate blood pressure and cholesterol. (use two to four)

****Reishi mushrooms - Great for cancer, lumps in the body, immune building, and detoxification. Helps with AIDS, high blood pressure, heart disease, Epstein-Barr, calming the mind, and improving memory. Raises our infection fighting T-cells. With cancers, I'd make these a must. Can be found at www.mountainroseherbs.com (use two to four)

****Red beets - Great for cancer, lumps in the body, and detoxifying man-made chemicals. Boosts the body's own detoxification enzymes and helps repair DNA. Beets should be added only *after* you've cleared the large majority of candida from your blood, so until you've stopped seeing lots of white stuff come out, it's best to hold off on beets. See Chapter 12 for more. (use one or two medium-sized red beets)

***Cilantro - Quickly and powerfully removes heavy metals. Great for preventing the brain damaging effects of heavy metals. Can be used regularly for about a month, and then less frequently. (use 1/4 to 1/2 cup)

***Seaweed - Removes accumulated radiation, and protected a lot of people after Hiroshima. Can be used regularly for two or three weeks, and then less frequently. Dulse, kombu, and wakame are great options. Before or after radiation exposure, it's a good idea to retain these. (use a 1/4 cup)

**Garlic - Great for candida, the heart, lowering blood pressure, and as a general anti-bacterial, anti-viral, and anti-parasitic agent. (use up to five cloves)

**Onion - Great for candida and an overall anti-bacterial, anti-fungal, and anti-parasitic agent. Start slowly with onion and build up. (use half to a whole medium-sized onion)

**Cabbage - Removes environmental estrogens, like the ones in plastic, that mimic our natural hormones and cause problems. Great for stubborn belly fat and cabbage also repairs our DNA. Use cabbage with caution because some people have cramping when they first start using it, however this generally goes away with more use. Start with small amounts and work up. Never retain an enema with cabbage. (use a small chunk up to a cup)

**Aloe vera - Powerful anti-inflammatory, soothing for the bowel, and a great detoxifier. The outer skin can be used or pealed first. (use one or two medium sized leaves)

**Oregano - Strong anti-bacterial, anti-fungal, and anti-parasitic agent with powerful antioxidant properties. (use up to two tablespoons at a time)

**Dandelion - Great for the liver and detoxification (use up to 10 big leaves and the roots too, if you have them)

*Turmeric - Helps the liver detoxify itself and is powerful for arthritis. A natural pain-killer and anti-inflammatory. But, be careful, it does stain. (use up to 2 tablespoons)

*Rosemary - Great for the nervous system; actually helps *rebuild* the nervous system which is key because many common chemicals damage our nervous systems. An anxiety reliever while also giving energy and improving memory. (use up to two tablespoons of the leaves)

*Burdock Root- Great for the liver and a blood purifier. Great for skin problems and liver problems. (use up to three tablespoons)

Powerful combos to try:

1) cilantro, seaweed and wild grass or greens 2) red beets and wild grasses or greens 3) mushrooms and wild grasses or greens 4) aloe, garlic, and wild grasses or greens 5) turmeric, rosemary and wild grasses or greens 6) dandelion, oregano and wild grasses or greens 7) cabbage, burdock root, and wild grasses or greens

Of course, but you're not limited to these combinations, so feel free to experiment and find and use what works best for you. Also, if you're cleansing long term, make sure you're rotating your enemas and greens to avoid overdoing any one type of plant. In addition, if you have a specific problem that other herbs are known to help with, I personally wouldn't hesitate to add those herbs to the coffee enemas either. Comfrey root is the only healing herb I'm familiar with that I wouldn't recommend adding to a coffee enema.

Wild grass is at the top of the list and it can be used in your green drinks too. It's discussed more in Appendix C, but essentially, wild grass is just that—grass you pick yourself that hasn't been fertilized or sprayed. Grass has all of the blood-building chlorophyll benefits of other greens, plus grass also contains another extremely powerful anti-cancer, detoxification, and strength building nutrient that isn't found many other places in nature, called CLA, or conjugated linoleic acid. The chlorophyll/CLA combination makes for some extremely powerful detoxification. If you can confirm that wheatgrass grown in trays doesn't have mold growing at the bottom, it's a form of grass that can be used too.

Coconut Oil

Coconut oil is used on this program as an implant enema (meaning it's retained in the body and not expelled), but

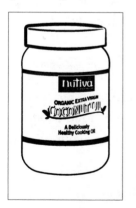

only *after* a coffee or coffee-based enema has first opened the bile ducts to the liver. Coconut oil is used after your bile ducts are open to encourage the oil to travel through your liver and be distributed into your bloodstream, where the oil can quickly and painlessly kill major amounts of candida as well as wipe out parasites, viruses, and bacteria. It's a very easy way to get major quantities of coconut oil in your system and it does a fabulous job of killing candida in between enema sessions. Actually, this technique has to be one of the fastest, most effective, and painless ways to remove candida en masse.

Chapter 9

Rules of the Game

Timing Your Cleanse

So, let's get down to business and look at the nuts and bolts of cleansing. Especially if you've never done any cleansing, you'll want to start your cleanse when life isn't hectic, or likely to be hectic. You'll need an hour or two each day for your enemas and just plain relaxing too. Plus, if a lot of this is new for you, it'll take a bit to get into the swing of things, but don't worry, as you get going, everything will become much more natural.

If finding time is an issue, many people can find the time for cleansing simply by turning off the television set. It's also a blessing to be away from the marketing of food products when you're changing your diet and upgrading your energy.

So, start your cleanse on a day when you're not working and you'll also want to buy all of your supplies before beginning, so if you have trouble finding something it won't be a problem. To make it easier, I now offer most of what you'll need on www.CleaningUpCleanse.com.

On Medication?

It's best not to take vitamins or medication during this program, so take only what is necessary. If you find yourself not needing medication or needing less during or after cleansing, work with a professional before making changes on your own, as simply eliminating some medications can be dangerous. Diabetics should also carefully monitor their insulin levels daily, as cleansing may significantly reduce the need for external insulin within a matter of days.

If you must take medication or birth control pills while cleansing, be sure not to take them two hours before or after a baking soda and psyllium drink, or before an enema. Those taking birth control should also use a backup method during this program and for three weeks afterward. Please note, however, that completely eliminating candida problems may be difficult while taking birth control. Birth control pills kill the healthy bacteria you'll be working to replace, and many kinds also elevate estrogen levels. Estrogen feeds the overgrowth and makes its elimination more difficult.

In addition, some drugs react with baking soda, either making them stronger or less effective, and a list of such known drugs is on p. 85. If you're taking any of these medications, you'll want to avoid using baking soda and consult the person who prescribed the medications you're taking if you have any questions.

Understand the Process;
Listen to Your Body

With this program, as in life, you are responsible for your health and well-being. So listen to your body. If you are tired, rest. If you are spacey, be careful and don't drive. Stand up slowly and make sure to keep your balance, especially after a bath. Exercise, particularly aerobic exercise and stretching, is encouraged—if you're up for it. Of course, avoid cigarettes, alcohol, and drugs, and if you need to quit smoking or other chemically addictive behaviors, see Ch. 12.

If you're very uncomfortable and the methods in the "Minimizing Detox Symptoms" chapter aren't helping, you may need to gently end your cleanse for a while. If you have fear, take things slowly, starting with small steps, to adjust to your comfort level. You'll also want to educate yourself before going into this. So, read the entire book and understand the process before beginning. Many people also benefit from reading it several times and keeping it handy while shopping for food and cleansing—especially if a lot of this information is new.

How Long to Cleanse?

The longer you cleanse, the deeper and more effective your cleanse will be. Since most people have been building toxicity since childhood, it's generally recommended to do fairly extensive cleansing to start, followed by regular maintenance in the years to come.

I believe that cleansing easily becomes needed by eighteen and honestly, I would have loved to have discovered cleansing at about fourteen. Younger individuals can also benefit from gentle and size-tailored versions of the cleanse, but under about twelve or fourteen, I'd only do that if a health problem or situation warrants it. However, that's unfortunately, that's becoming more common due to unnatural diets, antibiotic use, and what's become standard chemical-based living.

In any case, many adults will likely need several months of this type of deep cleansing to rid themselves of the bulk of their accumulation of toxicity and candida overgrowth. I wish I could say that the time required for deep cleansing is because these methods are slow, but the reality is that these methods are very quick and effective—much faster and more effective than other methods I've found.

The length of time needed is simply due to the amount of toxins the average person has stored. Of course, the length of time you'll need for thorough cleansing is entirely dependent upon the state of your body and how aggressively you cleanse—and it can be very different from person to person.

It's not uncommon for less toxic individuals to stop seeing large amounts of filth pouring out of them after a few months on this program. While this may not bring them entirely to the signs of complete cleanliness in the next section, it's an enormous step in the right direction. However, if you have a major candida problem with large pockets of waste, it will take you *considerably* longer than it will take someone who doesn't. If you have an extreme toxicity condition with stubborn pockets of waste, it can easily take a year *or longer* to cleanse thoroughly. In any case, if you're into cleansing for the long haul and the filth just keeps pouring out, it's best take some breaks during the process. So, take a few weeks off from the enemas every three months, just to give your body a rest.

It's also much better to do a few weeks of cleansing—even if your body needs more—than to do none at all. You can always do more later, and the key is often to just get started. Besides, once you get comfortable with cleansing and start to see and feel the benefits, you'll likely want to do more—even if you felt hesitant in the beginning. Believe it or not, I once was hesitant with cleansing too! And even though there's a lot of information in this book, applying it is rather simple once you get the hang of the key concepts.

So, if you're up for it, six weeks is a great start. But, if that's longer than you're up for, do what you're comfortable with. And if you're up for more, go for it. You can also pre-plan a time frame, or just cleansing until you feel like stopping, whatever works best for you.

In any case, using these enemas and massage, most people will see huge amounts of filth pouring out of them each day—so you'll know when you're finished and if you have work to do. People on the more toxic side sometimes wonder if the filth will ever stop pouring out of them. And, yes, actually, it does. It's just a matter of what all is in there. When it comes down to it, wouldn't you rather have this filth on the *outside* of you, rather than the inside, even if it does take a little while?

After the initial cleansing has removed many years of accumulated waste, it's wise to cleanse two or more weeks per
year, and follow the diet and lifestyle tips in Chapters 13
and 14. Your follow-up cleanses can be broken up or done
all at once—and if you're jumping back into cleansing after a break, you can start where you left off, as long you're
comfortable. If you haven't reached complete cleanliness but
are no longer up for aggressive cleansing, you can also make
cleansing part of your lifestyle, and add in a coffee-based enema every week or so, while following a diet from nature and
consuming lots of coconut oil and healthy bacteria.

Knowing When You're Candida- and Toxin-free

When you're absolutely candida- and toxin-free, you'll pass
the spit test several days in a row. In addition, your tongue,
front to back, will be light red, without the common white
coating. While it can definitely take some time and effort
to reach this stage, these are signs that your body is entirely free from toxicity. When you get there, it's unlikely that
you'll have any health problems, although most people start
dropping health problems *long* before they reach this stage.
It's also unlikely that you'll see large amounts of filth being
released from your body with the enemas, especially after
the first release or two in a session, which removes new accumulation.

It should be noted though, that there can be areas of the body that can be hard to reach with the enemas in this program. This is especially true if you have a lump, solid candida mass, or stubborn pocket of waste that you're having a hard time breaking down, or one an area that's not easily accessible by the massage—like your lungs, other organs, or sometimes the head/face area. In these instances, you may stop seeing large amounts of filth being released with the enemas, but you may not have a clear tongue or be passing the spit test. This is because the candida and filth are harder to reach.

At this point, coconut oil mini-fasting and juice fasting, particularly fasting on green juices, are your best bets to reach the rest of it and you can do either with the enemas in this book. Hydrogen peroxide skin cleansing is another extremely powerful method. (All in Chapter 12) Yet another option is to maintain the diet with lots of coconut oil, green drinks, and aerobic exercise, and come back to cleansing in a few weeks or months and see if your body is ready to remove more.

On the other hand, sometimes we may also need to understand that we can only do so much to turn around what, for many people, have been decades of poor eating and lifestyle habits, by the body's standards. If this is the case with you, focus on the filth that you have been able to remove—because if you're like most people, it will have been an enormous amount. Then, decide what you'd like to do. If some of the chemicals and toxins have severely damaged your organs, it may not be possible to bring them back completely, but it's certainly worth a try—and removing the root cause is always better than leaving it in there.

Safe for Everyone?

I believe these methods are very safe, and extremely health-giving. In fact, I believe that leaving your accumulated toxicity in your body is what's not safe. That said, there are some people who shouldn't cleanse, and others who shouldn't do a detoxification program without closer supervision.

Pregnant or nursing women should never cleanse, as they'd actually be feeding their toxins to their baby. However, before becoming pregnant is an excellent time to detoxify your body and doing so will provide a clean home for your baby and avoid transferring candida overgrowth to him or her, as commonly occurs when moms have the overgrowth. It's also advisable for fathers to cleanse before providing the seed for a child.

Since your liver and kidneys filter toxins from your body, it's important that they are functioning, so they can do this job effectively. Anyone with a serious or life-threatening illness, particularly of these organs, should cleanse very slowly and only under the guidance of a professional who has experience with detoxification programs. Releasing excessive toxicity quickly with damaged organs can harm the already strained organs.

Young children and older people, at a minimum, should use decreased amounts of all of the supplements, particularly the baking soda. Honestly though, I wouldn't suggest this cleansing program for children under twelve unless a health condition warranted it. I would, however, recommend the ongoing diet, chemical-free living, coconut oil, and plenty of healthy bacteria for children to avoid *creating* health conditions in them. Baking soda is never appropriate for infants.

Anyone with congestive heart failure should not use any baking soda in this cleanse. Baking soda also isn't appropriate for anyone on a doctor-prescribed low sodium diet or anyone with high blood pressure. Using baking soda is also cautioned for anyone with elevated blood sodium, low blood calcium, or problems with urination. If you're in these groups, you'll want to omit the baking soda in the drinks (at a minimum) and you may want to cleanse without using baking soda at all.

To cleanse without baking soda, simply leave it out of the psyllium drinks and substitute water enemas whenever baking soda enemas are called for. When baking soda is used in a coffee enema, just use a coffee enema with green juice instead. (Ch. 8, 10, and Ap. D)

If you have questions about the safety of cleansing with your particular situation, you should contact a naturally oriented health care provider. Unfortunately, most traditional medical doctors aren't educated about cleansing and how or why it works—and it's important that you get advice from someone who understands the process and why it's effective. If you have questions during cleansing, I offer some e-mail support included if you've purchased your cleansing supplies from www.CleaningUpCleanse.com. Other options are to check this book again as many questions are answered here, or do some research on the Internet to see if you can find the answer on your own. I also offer phone consultations, if they're needed.

In any case, if I had any health condition, extensive cleansing and superior nutrition are where I'd start—and a few years ago, I had so many large and small health problems I couldn't count them all on both hands. Cleansing extensively and providing superior nutrition are exactly what I did do, and are the reasons I've eliminated each of those problems. I'm also confident that deep and aggressive cleansing can help most people do the same for whatever problems that they face. Problems related to more toxicity, just take longer.

Drug Interactions

As we've talked about, using baking soda can react or interfere with some medications and if you are taking any of the drugs below, you should avoid using baking soda. Of course, if you have any questions, consult with the person who prescribed the medication and a professional familiar with detoxification methods.

Ketoconazole (Nizoral), lithium, chlorpropamide, methotrexate, tetracyclines, methenamine (Mandelamine), salicylates, amphetamines, anorexiants, mecamylamine, ephedrine, pseudoephedrine, flecainide, quinidine, quinine

Food Interactions

Those with gallstones, ulcers, heartburn, or stomach problems should avoid using dandelion. Those with epilepsy or seizure disorders should avoid using fennel. If you are taking any medication, avoid grapefruit and grapefruit juices; they can interfere with the medicine's ability to break down, which can be dangerous. While dairy isn't part of this program and it's recommended that baking soda shouldn't be taken near food, baking soda should never be taken near dairy; it can cause a reaction. Using beets, spinach, kale or parsley in quantity isn't appropriate for anyone with oxalate-based kidney stones. If you have these stones, I'd use wild grass for your green drinks and enemas instead. Using seaweed in quantity, in the veggie wraps or the enemas, also isn't recommended with hyperthyroidism. If you have soy allergies, you'll want to avoid using shoyu. In the veggie wraps a little sea salt can be substituted.

Chapter 10

Let's Do It! Step-by-Step Instructions

What you should know

The Cleaning Up! Cleanse is designed to be flexible, so whenever possible, there's room for personal taste and preference. Many different people will do *The Cleaning Up! Cleanse*, and some will have the time, energy, commitment, and resources to do more than others—and that's okay. It's important not to let relatively minor things block you from cleansing.

There's flexibility in how often you do the enemas, and you can cleanse as long as you desire—whether that's two weeks or until you're completely cleansed. You can modify the recipes provided, or create your own, as long as they're within the guidelines of acceptable foods. As we'll talk about, you can also speed up or slow down your cleanse to meet the needs of your body and your comfort level. A couple of sample days are provided, but they can be used as guides and they don't need to be followed exactly. However, if they work for you, they can be easy ways to fit everything in. But, you can absolutely modify the timing to your schedule and preferences. Aside from a few timing requirements with the baking soda and psyllium drinks, enemas, and probiotics, which are listed in this chapter, exactly when you do things isn't really important.

First and foremost, when doing a cleanse, it's important to remember that everyone comes from a different place. One might be an ex-smoker, overweight, and have a number of health problems. Another may have been a raw food vegetarian for the last fifteen years and has consciously avoided chemical contaminants. You'll need to make an effort to understand where you fall on this spectrum and adjust your cleanse to meet the needs of your body. If you think you might be on the more toxic side, just cleanse slower, especially in the beginning.

The perfect pace for one person may be too fast for another. And that's okay. The perfect length for one person may be too long for another. And that's okay, too. Your body needs what your body needs, and your job while cleansing is to listen to your body and adjust. Extreme detoxification symptoms are a sign that you're moving too quickly and it's best to at least temporarily slow your cleanse. So, remember, to slow your cleanse: eat more cooked foods, suspend your use of coconut oil, and just use the coffee enemas. Or, to speed your cleanse: simply eat entirely raw meals, have more green drinks, and use more coconut oil. There aren't upper limits to the amounts of coconut oil or green drinks you can have.

The Cleaning Up! Cleanse Involves:

✻ Eating foods and using recipes from *The Cleaning Up! Diet.*

✻ Consuming extra minerals each day—with fresh-squeezed or blended sweet, green juices.

✻ Consuming five or more tablespoons of coconut oil each day—in the coconut oil soups.

✻ Consuming one baking soda and psyllium drink each day.

✻ Doing specific enemas daily to clean your colon and entire body of impacted waste.

✻ Taking probiotics immediately after your enemas.

Each Step in Detail

✳ *Eating foods and using recipes from* The Cleaning Up! Diet.

This is done to avoid feeding candida and to allow your body to naturally begin cleansing. You're encouraged to eat as often and as much as you like, and until your hunger is satisfied. The salads, coconut oil soups, and green drinks should make up the bulk of your diet and if you're hungry, simply make larger portions or eat more often. In fact, you really shouldn't be hungry; it will make the whole process more difficult. While each day can certainly have some variance, one way to do this program is to have a large salad, coconut oil soup, and green drink each day (the second two are discussed more in just a minute). Then, just enjoy whatever else on the program you'd like to eat.

Those without candida issues or sugar sensitivities can include with moderation fresh fruit, fresh fruit juices, organic corn, beets, and fresh vegetable juices made with carrots or beets. Either way, always keep appropriate foods on hand, such as carrots, tomatoes, or avocados with some of the salad dressings, to snack on if you are hungry.

You'll also be taking in extra enzymes and heathy bacteria by consuming a cup or two of raw, unpasteurized sauerkraut each week. The kraut can be added to your salads, your soups with coconut oil (after they've been blended), or just eaten straight. *The Cleaning Up! Cleanse diet* is outlined in Chapter 7 and the recipes to use are in Appendices B and C.

✳ *Consuming extra minerals each day with deliciously sweet green juices.*

Your body needs four alkaline minerals (also called electrolytes) to function properly and be in balance. These minerals are sodium, potassium, magnesium, and calcium. Baking soda is largely composed of the alkaline mineral sodium. It's a form of sodium that can be used by your body—which is different from table salt (which is toxic).

However, doing liver cleansing and using baking soda can decrease the amounts of other minerals in your body, so while cleansing, you'll want to consume lots of mineral-rich foods. Mineral-rich foods are easy to add to your diet and you'll do it with the daily consumption of fresh squeezed or blended juices, especially with hearty green drinks.

Some of the best mineral sources: Wild grass, spinach, parsley, Swiss chard, collard greens, butter lettuce, cabbage, dandelion, kale, beet greens, and celery.

So, to add extra minerals to your body, have one or more fresh-squeezed or blended juices each day and rely heavily on the green juices. In addition to being mineral-rich, the green drinks are incredibly detoxifying and you'll be using the sweet herb stevia to make sure they're sweet and delicious. Because you're going to be doing so much work on your liver, using dandelion as a liver tonic regularly is strongly recommended too. (Drink recipes, Appendix C).

✱ Consuming five or more tablespoons of coconut oil each day—in the coconut oil soups.

You'll use coconut oil orally to start killing the candida in your intestines and begin detoxifying your entire body. Coconut oil also helps raise the metabolism for those with weight to lose and helps maintain weight for those without weight to lose. The more coconut oil you take in, the shorter your candida elimination time will be. But because it's so powerful, coconut oil can cause detox symptoms. So, move slowly in increasing your consumption of coconut oil, especially if you think you might be on the more toxic side.

Coconut oil is used as your primary cooking oil, and it's also used liberally in the dressings and soups. On this program, it's great to have the coconut oil soups each day while using increasing amounts of the oil. These soups are an easy way to take in concentrated doses of the oil which enhances the detoxification process considerably. So, start by having soups with one to two tablespoons a day during the first week, then add a tablespoon or two per day, each week thereafter—and aim to maintain at five tablespoons or more per day in the soups. If you don't make it to the high end consistently, it's okay. Just use what you're comfortable with—and if you want to add in even more, that's okay too. For even more detoxification power, you can have these soups twice a day. However, if you are detoxifying too rapidly and feeling uncomfortable, introduce the oil even more slowly. Or, if you can hardly feel a thing, step up the pace and add it in more rapidly.

In addition, you can use as much coconut oil in the salad dressings, vegetable wrap dressings, and other recipes as you like. With coconut oil and cleansing, as long as it's not causing uncomfortable detoxification symptoms, the more the better. Actually, as long as any detoxification symptoms aren't extreme, they're not a problem for your body, but because this program is designed to be done while working, this is where they might cause a problem. In addition, if you're experiencing detoxification symptoms with these soups, especially tiredness, try having them a little before bed, so you can just sleep though them.

In any case, if you take in a bunch of coconut oil and feel uncomfortable, rest and an enema are the quickest remedies. Taking psyllium after having lots of coconut oil will do two things: 1) speed the candida out of your small intestine (a good thing!) and 2) possibly cause intestinal cramping and tiredness as this is happening. I like to do this on occasion for the benefits of cleaning out the small intestine—but only when I can sleep afterward.

At times, you may also feel you've overdosed on coconut oil, and you may well have. It's an interesting phenomenon that if we overdo even healthy foods, they will taste bad to us until our body needs the nutrients in them again. So, if the oil begins tasting awful to you, stop consuming it until it becomes palatable again. Sometimes this takes a week or so and it can take a month or longer, if you've really used a lot for a while. However, even if the coconut oil tastes awful, if you are using it in the enemas, you can continue to do so for powerful candida killing and detoxification. And know that during this program, especially if you're cleansing longer term, there will likely be times you'll need to take breaks from the coconut oil.

This flavor-changing phenomenon actually occurs more often when we're eating foods from nature, and it's also a good reason to vary your salads, green juices, and soups too, to avoid over-doing any particular veggies. If you're taking a break from coconut oil, you may also want to take a break from the soups and have more of the salads, vegetable wraps, and green drinks instead to avoid this with your favorite coconut oil soup ingredients. And with any food, if this flavor change occurs, it's time to hold off on that food for a while, until it tastes good again.

✳ *Consuming one baking soda and psyllium drink each day.*

The baking soda and psyllium drinks are an oxygen-rich scrubbing solution for your entire intestinal track. The baking soda also helps oxygenate and alkalize your entire body to create an environment which candida and many pathogens don't thrive and often have a hard time existing. Because baking soda neutralizes the acidic waste you'll be releasing—or it turns the waste into less harmful compounds—baking soda also helps make sure you feel well on your cleanse.

Because baking soda can react with some substances and psyllium can absorb substances consumed before or after it, you should have your juices, food, and supplements at least one hour before or after these drinks. If you're taking any medication, leave at least two hours on either side of each drink. To speed and enhance your intestinal cleansing, particularly if you find the psyllium isn't moving through your system, you can also have two cups of senna tea each day, but only for one week each month. Senna tea acts as a natural herbal laxative.

The recipe for this sweet and believe it or not, very decent tasting drink is in Appendix C. If you're cleansing long-term, after three months end your use of oral baking soda and just have psyllium with stevia instead, or just use baking soda occasionally. If you're cleansing short-term (under a month), try having two of these drinks each day, unless you want to cleanse slower.

If you have low levels of hydrochloric acid and are concerned about drinking baking soda, you can have the Cinnamon and Spice Tea with cayenne pepper (p. 214) thirty minutes before each meal. The cayenne pepper will raise your levels of hydrochloric acid and a touch of cayenne can also be deliciously added to other herbal teas too.

✳ *Doing specific enemas daily to cleanse your colon, liver, and entire body of impacted waste, while alkalizing your body and removing candida and other pathogens.*

Colon cleansing can be done any time of the day and to speed your cleanse, it can be done twice a day—as long as you're up for it. The enema schedule is later in this chapter, the recipes are in Appendix D, and the instructions to give yourself an enema are in Chapter 11. The general rules are to wait at least an hour after a big meal and to always replenish your healthy bacteria immediately afterward. It's also best not to do your enemas within two hours after a coconut oil soup, to make sure you're utilizing as much of the oil as possible.

✶ *Taking probiotics immediately after your enemas.*

Have one serving of probiotics immediately after any enema session to replenish your healthy bacteria. Then, be sure not to consume anything except water or green juice for thirty minutes after your probiotics to give them time to implant. Your healthy bacteria are also replenished in this cleanse with the regular use of sauerkraut in your meals. If desired, you can also have two-thirds of a cup of raw sauerkraut after each enema to replenish your healthy bacteria instead of taking probiotic supplements. If you skip the kraut in your meals, you'll also need to take an extra serving of probiotics each day, just before bed.

Anything Else?

While using baking soda in the drinks and enemas provides a great deal of the power in this program, you'll also want to avoid having high levels of oxygen in your blood for an extended period of time, which is why you'll stop consuming baking soda orally after three months, or just use it occasionally after this point. You'll also need to be aware of the signs of becoming overly alkaline so you can cut back on baking soda, orally and in the enemas, if they occur.

The most prominent signs of becoming overly alkaline are being very tired and lethargic (although sometimes this just happens with deep cleansing too), and also having very shallow breath. You may even notice that you're subconsciously holding your breath for a few seconds, between breaths.

You'll actually want to watch for the shallow breath and if it occurs, cut back on or end your use of baking soda for at least 72 hours to give your body the space to normalize itself and release some of the excess oxygen. You can also help your body along by holding your breath, which keeps extra carbon dioxide in your body and neutralizes the oxygen. Or, if desired, you can eat some acid forming foods, like beans or lentils, to speed the process along too. At this point, you may want to discontinue using any oral baking soda, if you're using it, and scale back on the amount you're using in your enemas too, while watching your breath before using more. Generally, the baking soda in the enemas is fairly immediately released, so it's not likely to be a problem, but still, it's something you should be aware of.

Also, those under age eighteen, the elderly, and those in weak condition will want to reduce the supplements, coconut oil, and enema doses and concentrations considerably to make the process more comfortable. Children, due to their size difference, and the elderly, due to the fact that they may have a compromised ability to excrete excess oxygen, should reduce the amount of baking soda by half or more.

The Cleaning Up! Cleanse: Sample Day One

* *First Thing in the Morning* - Have a baking soda and psyllium drink. (Appendix C).

* *Snack* - An hour after your psyllium drink, have a fresh squeezed or blended green juice. (Appendix C) Alternatively, have some vegetable wraps using coconut oil in the dressing. (Appendix B)

* *Lunch* - Have a big salad. Use a blended dressing and nuts, if you're using them. (Appendix B)

* *Snack* - Two hours after lunch, have a fresh squeezed or blended green juice. (Appendix C) Alternatively, have some herbal mushrooms (Appendix B) or a cup of raw sauerkraut.

* *Early Evening Enema* - Do a two-gallon enema using the stages to determine which kind to do. After your enema take 10 to 25 billion probiotic microorganisms, orally. (Stages, pp. 100 - 104, Recipes, Appendix D)

* *Dinner* - Thirty or more minutes after your probiotics have a blended soup with coconut oil. If desired, have your soup over chopped vegetables. (Appendix C)

The Cleaning Up! Cleanse: Sample Day Two

* **First Thing in the Morning** - Do a two-gallon enema using the stages to determine which kind to do. After your enema take 10 to 25 billion probiotic microorganisms, orally. (Stages, pp. 100- 104, Recipes, Appendix D)

* **30 min. after your probiotics** - Have a large blended soup with coconut oil. Alternatively, have a large salad. (Appendix B)

* **Lunch** - Have a large salad with a blended dressing— or a large blended soup with coconut oil. (Appendix B)

* **Snack** - Two hours after lunch, have a fresh squeezed or blended green juice. (Appendix C) If you're including nuts, have a small handful of raw, soaked nuts with sea salt. (Soaking nuts, Appendix E)

* **Dinner** - Have some vegetable wraps, a large vegetable saute, or another large salad with a blended coconut oil dressing. (Appendix B)

* **An hour or more after dinner** - Have a baking soda drink and psyllium drink. (Appendix C).

The Cleaning Up! Cleanse—The Order

The Cleaning Up! Cleanse introduces the enemas in an order which allows for cleansing that the body will support without going into overload. Each enema stage produces different effects and builds on the previous one, so it's important to do them in order. You'll clean your colon before you clean your liver. Then you'll detoxify your liver before moving into the heavier Stages III, IV, and V cleansing. This is done to ensure you don't induce massive detoxification before your pathways for removal are open, and your body is ready to handle it.

Stage I is just three days long and Stages II through IV are each a week long. Then, you can stay in Stage V as long as you need or want before ending your cleanse. If you want to cleanse slower, you can stay in Stages II, III, or IV longer, before moving on. Or, if you've done a bunch of colon and liver cleansing previously, you might want to start in Stage III, or advance through the stages more quickly. If you aren't seeing large amounts of filth being removed with the enemas, it's uncommon, but it does happen occasionally. If this is the case, I encourage you to advance to the next enema stage. It may be that there isn't much filth in there, but it's more likely that it's just a little stuck and it can take some time to loosen it.

In Appendix D, you'll find the recipes to prepare your enema solutions, and the amounts to use for the herbal and vegetable coffee enemas are in Chapter 8.

You can do the enemas once or twice a day and the more often you do them, the faster and more thorough your cleansing will be. But do what you're comfortable with. If you need to take breaks or do them less frequently because of your schedule or other reasons—feel free to do so. However, because the enemas help remove the filth the rest of the program will be loosening, you'll feel much better during the process if you do the enemas frequently, especially in the beginning. Of course, you'll become much cleaner too. On the other hand, if you're up for more aggressive cleansing you can use an extra gallon of the coffee-based enema solution in your sessions. Just make another gallon, using the same proportions. If you're up for it—it's recommended—particularly if there's considerable filth still pouring out of you at the end of the session.

If you're cleansing longer-term and after your colon is relatively clean, you can also drop the baking soda pre-coffee enemas and move straight into the coffee-based enemas instead. You'll know when you reach this point when the baking soda pre-coffee enemas are no longer removing a considerable amount of filth, except perhaps some with the first release. However, if you do this, just retain your first enema in the session about 30 seconds (instead of six minutes), so that any new accumulation is quickly released and doesn't travel with the coffee into your liver. Doing this can make your enemas considerably faster or if you want, you can also use one and a half or two gallons of a coffee-based enema solution instead of one gallon, for deeper detoxification. Just increase the recipes proportionally.

Stage I

Stage I uses baking soda enemas to clean your colon and remove candida from your large intestine. Cleaning your colon is important in and of itself and it's also critical to ensure an open pathway out of the body for the toxicity you'll be removing in the later stages.

The Methods:

✴ Do one or two enema sessions each day. Use a two-gallon baking soda enema. Follow each enema session with probiotics.

Stage II

Stage II uses coffee enemas to clean your liver. It's important that your liver is cleansed so that it can filter and effectively remove the filth you're going to dislodge in Stages III, IV, and V.

The Methods:

✴ Do one or two enema sessions each day. Use a one-gallon baking soda enema first, then a one-gallon coffee enema. Follow each enema session with probiotics.

Stage III

Stage III uses coffee and baking soda enemas to cleanse your liver while alkalizing your entire body and quickly dislodging and removing candida and filth en masse from all areas of your body.

The Methods:

✱ Do one or two enema sessions each day. Use a one-gallon baking soda enema first, then a one-gallon coffee/baking soda enema. Follow each enema session with probiotics.

Stage IV

In Stage IV, you'll add greens to your coffee and baking soda enemas for even more powerful detoxification. For greens, you can use either wild grasses (more in Appendix C) or store bought greens like parsley, kale, or spinach. If you're up for picking them, wild grasses are preferred because they're more powerful detoxifiers. You can also add any of the detoxifying or healing foods and herbs in Chapter 8 to these enemas for more power and to address specific problems.

The Methods:

✱ Do one or two enema sessions daily. Use a one- gallon baking soda enema first, then a one-gallon coffee, baking soda, green juice and herbal enema. Follow each enema session with probiotics.

Stage V

Stage V is the same as Stage IV, however, you'll now use the coconut oil implant enemas as the final enema in your enema session. Using coconut oil will turbo-charge your candida elimination and greatly speed your detoxification.

The Methods:

✱ Do one or two enema sessions each day. Use a one-gallon baking soda enema first, then a one-gallon coffee, baking soda and green juice enema.

✱ Follow your coffee, baking soda and green juice enema with a coconut oil retention enema. After inserting the oil, follow the protocols on pp. 118-119 to bring the oil to your liver to do its magic. Follow each enema session with probiotics. If you're doing two enema sessions a day, just use coconut oil in the later one.

✱ Instead of using coconut oil, you can alternatively retain a half cup or so of the Stage IV enemas and release in an hour or two, when you feel the need to release. If you're going to retain these, you'll want to leave out the baking soda, however. You can also toggle between retaining the Stage IV enemas and using the coconut oil retention enema, or just use what works best for you.

Ending Your Cleanse

You can end your cleanse when you have removed all of the candida and toxicity from your body, or are otherwise ready to end your cleanse. To end your cleanse, you'll need to transition to your ongoing diet and substantially rebuild the healthy bacteria in your colon. As you know, having hearty healthy bacteria in your colon can prevent many problems.

The Methods:

* Adopt the transition diet, as outlined below.
* Consume at least ten billion probiotic microorganisms daily for three months past cleansing. For added protection, consume two or more cups of unpasteurized sauerkraut each week too.
* Occasionally, people have problems resuming regular bowel function after extensive use of enemas, and if that happens with you, drink lots water each day and have a cup of senna tea in the evening, the later for only one week each month. Aerobic exercise and occasional psyllium drinks also help move things along, but generally, it doesn't take long.

Diet Transitioning

Many people use cleansing to kick-start healthier long-term eating and many people find that once they've removed considerable amounts of toxicity, the cravings for meat, processed food, and junk foods disappear—making it an ideal time to make the change. Especially when you begin experiencing the spiritual benefits that have long been connected with cleansing and eating nature's foods, I hope that eating only nature's foods will become a lifelong habit for you. However, if your diet is going to be significantly different than it was on the cleansing program, transition to it slowly—particularly to the more processed, sugared, and less natural foods. And if you've just gotten rid of a major candida problem, I wouldn't recommend going back to a high sugar or processed carbohydrate diet.

In any case, Chapter 13 will help you upgrade your on-going diet with simple healthy tips and Appendix E will get you get started with some more simple, delicious recipes.

✶ If you were cleansing for candida and it hasn't been eliminated (you can tell by spit testing), it's wise to follow *The Cleaning Up! Cleanse diet* and continue taking coconut oil and probiotics until you're ready to cleanse again.

✶ It's also a good idea to keep the salads, coconut oil, and green drinks in your diet while transitioning, and ideally long-term.

✶ Begin enjoying raw, soaked nuts and nut milks regularly to help your body rebuild—especially if you've cleansed extensively. (Appendix E)

✶ When you've finished cleansing for candida, add sweet and carbohydrate-rich foods back in *slowly*. Start by adding fruit, beans, nuts, seeds, and whole grains, including brown rice, wild rice, and quinoa. It's best to keep sugar, refined carbohydrates, unhealthy oils, and red meats out of your diet for at least two or three months after cleansing, and ideally permanently.

Chapter 11

Giving Yourself an Enema—Relax, It's Not That Hard!

The first thing you want to do is relax! If you've never given yourself an enema, I promise, it's not as hard or scary as it seems. Remember, almost everyone is scared of the enemas in the beginning, but after a couple, just about everyone says they really weren't that bad. And they do get easier as you get used to them. *So, relax!* Turn on some music to listen to while you're doing your enemas. You'll be fine!

Preparation

First of all, you'll prepare your solutions as described in Appendix D and bring them with you to the bathroom in your glass jugs. Then, you'll lay a large, old towel on your bathroom floor, or in the tub, if the floor isn't big enough for you to lie down comfortably. You'll be lying on the towel, so it should be thick enough to keep you comfortable and old

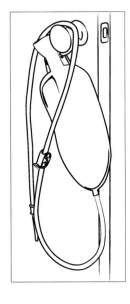

enough so that if some of the solution spills, you won't care.

Next, if your enema bag isn't already assembled, you want to assemble it according to the instructions with your kit. This generally means attaching the hose to the bag, sliding the on/off switch up the hose, then twisting the insertion tip onto the other end of the hose. That's it. You're all done.

Now, just pour the appropriate solution into your bag. But, before pouring, make sure the clamp is in the closed position because if it isn't closed, the solution will come out before you're ready. That can be messy, so be sure to check. After the bag is full, you'll want to hold the tip over a drain and open the clamp for a few seconds to let out a little of the solution. This will let the air out of the tube and avoid filling you up with air.

Using the hook provided, you'll now hang your enema bag on a towel rack or doorknob, about three feet in the air. If you hang it much higher, the solution will come out too quickly for comfort and if you hang it much lower, there won't be enough pressure.

Now, strip down and make yourself comfortable. You can use a space heater if you want to keep warm, but keep it a good distance away from your enema bag in case of a spill. Listening to music is great too and highly recommended.

Lube Up and Insert

Now, just pour a small amount of a vegetable oil, like olive or coconut oil, onto a wad of toilet paper and wipe some oil onto the tip being inserted. Then, wipe your rear with the oiled tissue too, to make insertion easy and painless. And have no fear! Only the oiled tip, which is about the diameter of a straw and just a couple inches long, is inserted.

Now, lie down on your back on the towel, with your knees bent. Then, holding the hose near the tip, reach behind you and gently insert the tip. Be sure not to shove it, but guide it in gently. Twisting it slightly makes insertion easier, as does deep breathing and tilting your pelvis slightly up. Just relax and take your time.

Fill Slowly, Massage Your Stomach

Once the tip is inserted, release the clamp to let the solution flow in slowly and know that you can stop the flow of solution at any time by simply closing the clamp. Be sure to do so if you need to and take your time and don't fill too quickly.

Holding the clamp in one hand, you'll also begin massaging your stomach with the other hand to help loosen the debris and break up air pockets. Begin your massage at the lower left-hand side of your abdomen, and move your hand counterclockwise up the left side of your abdomen, across the top of your abdomen (under your rib cage), and down the right side. This will help loosen the impacted fecal matter for its release. Massaging your stomach in this manner is important for the first couple of weeks of enemas, but as the filth from your colon is removed, you can transition to the massage techniques discussed later in this chapter.

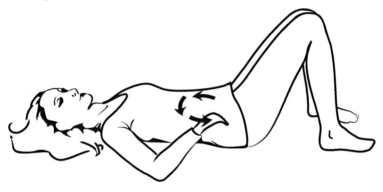

Release and Repeat…

When you feel full, or the need to release, just close the clamp on the hose to stop the flow of solution. For enemas that you retain for a few minutes, just lie there and relax. Then, when you need to release, remove the tip and go to the toilet to do so. Most people can take the contents of one-third to one, two-quart enema bag before needing to release, but only you can know how much is right for you.

Now, just stay on the toilet until everything has been expelled and sometimes this takes a few minutes. While releasing, you can massage your colon the opposite way from when you were filling. Start at the bottom right, move up the right side, across the top under the ribs, and down the left side. This will encourage a release. Don't be alarmed if there is occasional cramping when on the toilet; it means that an unusually toxic load is coming. Just be patient and stay on the toilet until it does and when you see it, you'll know what I'm talking about!

Then, repeat the process as many times as it takes to use all of your solution(s), which will entail refilling the bag, and yourself, several times. During a single session, you can fill and release ten or more times. If you are filling and releasing considerably fewer than eight times, you may want to increase the amount of total solution you are using. Also, be sure to lubricate the tip and your rear before each insertion to assure your comfort. And it's a good idea to close the toilet seat before flushing and keep it closed when filling up, as quite a bit of spray comes out of the toilet after flushing.

Flipping, Squeezing, Massaging, and Stretching

One of the most important things you can do while the enemas are inside of you—and this is particularly important with enemas using coffee—is to *stretch and squeeze* all of your muscles and body parts. It's hard to overemphasize the importance of these techniques. These methods will loosen the toxicity and candida throughout your body and are critical to making candida problems a thing of the past once it's left your colon. The massage can physically break up your pockets of waste too, and make the waste corralled in them available for removal.

During the first two enema stages, with the baking soda enemas inside of you, flip onto your stomach and lie on each side to remove the candida from all sides of your colon walls.

While holding the Stage III, IV and V coffee-based enemas inside you, massage, squeeze, and stretch your feet, hands, shoulders, neck, calves, bottom, arms, face, back, and hips—essentially all areas of your body—as hard as you comfortably can. Seek out and target any areas with pain, knots, tightness, or discomfort. Most areas with soreness or tightness are areas with toxicity that you can now remove, and you may be surprised at how many sore areas, including sore muscles, you find.

Then, stretch like you would in a stretching class. Bring your knees to your chest and hold them there. Cross one foot over the other bent knee and bring them to your chest. Cross one arm over your chest and place a hard massage ball underneath your shoulder and upper back muscles being stretched. Kneel with your head to the ground to bring blood to your upper body. While in this position, arch your back and bring your head backward.

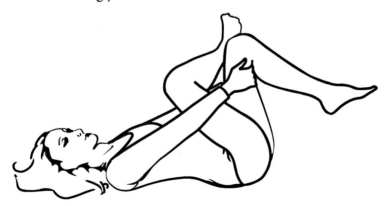

Stretch your neck by bringing your chin to your chest and tilt your head as far as it will reach toward each shoulder. Use your knuckles to break up the filth stored in your throat and neck. You can also massage your abdomen to break up filth in your small intestine. I've also found that dark moles are often markers of areas with large amounts of toxic filth underneath, so be sure to massage these areas well. With dark moles, I actually think we're just seeing the filth come out—through the skin.

You can also do stretches while sitting or standing after you've allowed any coffee solution time to travel into your liver. While standing, you can clasp your hands behind your back and pull them up over your head. To reach your feet, ankles and the backs of your calves, it's helpful to sit up, with your legs folded underneath you (and your feet under your rear) and sit back on your feet. This is particularly helpful if you regularly have cold feet, which might be indicative of a lot of filth stored in your lower extremities. Sitting in lotus position (with the soles of your feet up) for a few minutes can be helpful too. When you're on the toilet, you can also massage your legs, feet, and calves.

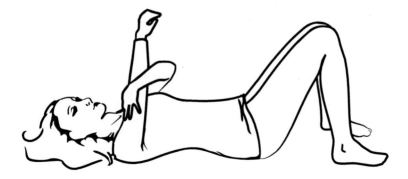

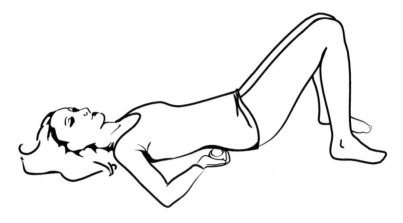

Doing sit ups with the coffee enemas inside of you can aid in the removal of filth from your back, spine, shoulders, and neck; just make sure you've given the coffee solution a few minutes to enter your liver before beginning. Find other stretches and positions that work for you, and *do them.*

Lying on a strategically placed massage ball can effectively remove the toxicity from the muscles of your shoulders, spine, shoulder blades, and lower back—areas so many people have problems with. If you're like me, you'll see huge releases of candida and toxicity from these areas and for a lot of people, this may be the key to saying good-bye to chronic back pain.

I've listed a lot of different stretches here, but don't worry, you don't need to do them all at once. Actually, I find it best to concentrate the massage on one or two areas per enema and that way, when you see the release, you'll know where it came from. Areas with a great deal of waste should be deeply massaged and stretched during repeated enema sessions until the knots or pain are gone and the release is free of candida and filth—and you may find areas with extreme amounts of waste that require several weeks or longer to re-move all of the waste. It took me *many* weeks (many months really) to break up the pockets of waste in my shoulders, neck, and throat, and to remove all of the candida and filth tightly packed in there. Some stubborn pockets of waste won't budge without relatively deep pressure and sometimes repeated deep pressure.

If you are trying to reach known pockets of waste or prob-lem areas, also be mindful of how gravity affects blood flow and position yourself to encourage blood flow to these areas. For example, if you have a lump on your left side, you might want to lie on your left, and position yourself so the area is as close to the ground as possible. However, before chang-ing positions, give the coffee-based solution a few minutes to travel into your liver.

You'll also see the candida you're removing—whitish, cot-ton-ball-like matter that generally floats is candida leaving your body. *Congratulations!* Candida can also have a yellow-ish or brownish tint if it's older and you may see strands, plastic-wrap-like sheets, or root-like structures being elimi-nated. My own body released it all—including clumps the size of golf balls, roots more than a foot long, and roots the size of my thumbs in diameter.

You'll also know when you've broken up a pocket of filth. Not only will the release be enormous and generally smelly, but the knot or soreness in that area will either have de-creased or been eliminated.

When You're Done...

When you're finished, it's nice to take a shower to relax and clean your external body. But, before jumping into the shower, clean up a bit. Rinse the inside of your enema bag with hot water and hang the bag to dry (so the water drips out). Rinse the containers you've used to hold the enema solutions with hot water too, and if you want to clean your enema bag more thoroughly, use a solution of hydrogen peroxide and water every week or so.

Cramping?

Occasionally, you may feel some cramping. If so, check to be sure the water you used wasn't cold, as cold water can cause cramping. If the cramping disappears after your release, it was caused by the filth in your system being dislodged. That (now mobile) toxic matter was making you ill, so be glad it's out of your body.

If cramping is severe or the enemas are extremely uncomfortable (two uncommon occurrences), you may want to stop doing the at-home enemas until you've had three or four professional colonics to clear a large portion of the debris.

How Long Will It Take?

Generally speaking, a two-gallon enema session (the amount recommended in this program) takes ninety minutes to two hours. So, give yourself some time; it's worth it. If you're short on time, even a quick one-gallon session is preferable to none. As your colon becomes cleaner and you no longer need the pre-coffee enema, you can drop that enema or replace it with more of a coffee-based enema. If you leave it out, you can cut the amount of time needed, in about half.

How Long to Keep the Enemas In?

Baking soda and water enemas can be retained in the body two minutes, but it's not necessary to hold them in longer.

Enemas with coffee are retained in the body about six minutes—to allow all of the blood in your body to travel through your liver and be cleansed. If you feel the need to expel before then, by all means do so. Feeling the need to release often means that something toxic has been dislodged—and you should let it out of your body.

Coconut oil enemas are retained in the body as long as possible, preferably overnight. They're used after enemas with coffee to send the coconut oil into your liver and throughout your body. Some people are concerned that the oil might harden in their bodies, but this is impossible. Coconut oil is liquid over 76 degrees, and the human body maintains a temperature of approximately 98.6 degrees. You'll actually see the oil released, undigested, the next day, usually with a bunch of other filth too.

The last half cup of your green and herbal coffee enema can also be retained for an hour or two, in lieu of the coconut oil. If you're retaining these, leave out the baking soda and release when needed.

Coconut Oil Enema Positions

With the coconut oil enemas, it's important that the oil reaches your liver to do its job. So, your liver is under your right rib cage and there are couple of ways to ensure the oil reaches your liver: 1) while lying on your back, bend your knees and lift your hips for 30 seconds—to bring the oil to the top of your colon—then roll over onto your right side and lie there for ten minutes or 2) while lying on your back, bend your knees and lift your hips for 30 seconds—to bring the oil to the top of your colon—then quickly flip over onto your knees and bend so that your head touches the ground. After 30 seconds in this position, bring your right shoulder to the ground, and lift your left shoulder into the air and hold this position for 30 seconds to bring the oil to the right side of your colon, and then resume the original head to ground position for about ten minutes. The goal with either of these methods is bring the oil to the top right-hand side of your colon, where it can be easily taken up by your liver.

Maintaining this position for about ten minutes will give the oil time to travel into your liver where it can do its phenomenal job of killing candida and pathogens throughout your

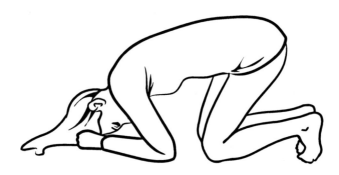

body. Making sure you give the coconut oil enough time to travel into your liver will also help avoid unwanted leakage, by ensuring that little of it remains in your colon. It may take a few days for your body to adjust to the coconut oil, but leakage is *not* common. However, if you have a problem with it, you may want to use less coconut oil. One caution, however: If you need to pass gas when using the coconut oil enemas, particularly when you first begin using them, you'll definitely want to do so over a toilet to avoid any surprises.

You can also use these positions with your coffee solutions, however for most people, as long as you've used enough solution, lying on your back will be just fine for your coffee-based enemas. Occasionally, people also have trouble retaining the coconut oil and one trick is to jog in place for a few minutes *before* inserting the oil. This will encourage a release to make sure you're eliminating all that needs to be eliminated before using the oil.

When using the coconut oil enemas, you can also try sleeping on alternate sides, if you sleep on your side. Your body does much of its regularly cleansing when you're asleep (and not digesting food), and the side that's on the mattress generally gets the most attention due to the way gravity affects blood flow. If you regularly sleep on one side, the side you don't sleep on may be in need of extra cleansing and this is a simple, way to do it. If you have any problems in the body in known locations, try sleeping (or at least spending several hours) with that area on the mattress. For a simple technique, it's very effective.

Coconut Oil Enemas—
Special Instructions

When doing the coconut oil enemas, you'll also want to hang your enema bag higher than three feet from the floor. Coconut oil is thicker than water, and at only three feet, several tablespoons of the oil will be left in the bag. I find it best to hang the bag as high as you can, while still being able to do the insertion. Good places to hang it can be a higher towel rack, the shower head, or a clothes hook. Or you can purchase a stick-on hook to hang it at the appropriate height.

After your coconut oil enema, you'll want to drain the excess oil from the bag into a container for disposal, instead of down your drain. You'll want as little of the oil as possible to go down your drains to protect them from the coconut oil cooling and solidifying in the pipes. (If this happens, just run hot water for a few minutes to melt the oil). Then, after removing the excess oil, rinse your bag with hot water to clear any remaining oil and prevent the oil from turning solid in your bag. This makes your next enema session easier, and protects your enema bag from developing leakage problems. If you don't rinse out the excess oil, you may need to run your bag under hot water for several minutes to melt the oil before your next enema session.

Chapter 12

Super-charge Your Cleanse

I've designed *The Cleaning Up! Cleanse* to be as simple and doable as possible. I know that a cleanse that's too complex will turn some people off, yet there will be others who are up for more. This section offers methods to "Super-charge Your Cleanse" your cleanse if you're up for doing them and also some methods just to address common problems, cleansing or not. So, just rotate these in as needed or desired but some of these methods, you'll want to incorporate in only after you've been cleansing for a little while to ensure your body can remove the junk you're going to be loosening.

Coconut Oil Skin Cleansing

Your skin, your largest organ, needs detoxification and coconut oil is a great everyday solution. Using coconut oil on your skin kills candida and bacteria in and underneath your skin, and can reach and remove candida in otherwise difficult to reach areas. Plus, coconut oil is highly moisturizing and amazing for general skin care. So, for daily use, simply use coconut oil instead of lotion and apply it after bathing and toweling dry. Just use a light layer, let it absorb for a few minutes, and then towel off again to remove the excess before dressing. It's best to do this head to toe; however, women should avoid using coconut oil on the face if they're putting makeup on afterward, as the oil will draw the makeup into the skin.

For problems above the neck, using coconut oil on your scalp is important too. So, find a few parts in your hair and rub in a couple tablespoons after evening showers. Then, let it soak in and wash your hair in the morning. As a bonus, coconut oil is a wonderful hair conditioner, but protect your clothes and pillow, as coconut oil does stain. If you have a great deal of toxicity in your head area, you may feel a bit out of it when using coconut oil on your face and scalp but this will pass as the area becomes cleaner.

Hydrogen Peroxide Skin Cleansing

For even more power, twice a week you can use some 3% hydrogen peroxide on your skin after you've applied some coconut oil. The coconut oil will pull the oxygen-rich hydrogen peroxide into your body to oxygenate it and reach areas of candida and filth that you're having trouble reaching with other methods. This is actually an extremely powerful and easy way to address candida and filth that's near the skin and harder to reach with the enemas. It's also great for battling colds, flus, and viral infections. In fact, it's so powerful that many of you, especially if you think you might be on the more toxic side, will want to dilute your 3% hydrogen peroxide in half using water, the first few times you do this. And it's best if you've cleansed three or more weeks before adding it in.

So, to do this, just lube up with a light layer of coconut oil and then sit in the tub and slowly pour a little hydrogen peroxide over yourself and rub it in deeply. Use hand-sized cupfuls and rub it in, before adding more.

You can use anywhere from eight to sixteen ounces of hydrogen peroxide each time, and if you're on the larger side, you can use more. Then, spend ten minutes rubbing it in, while you're sitting on some and reapplying what you've already applied and spilled. When you're done, just towel off and if you can, take a walk to get your blood moving. It's also important to wipe down the tub afterward. If not, it will be very slippery for the next person who bathes, so wipe it down well to prevent an accident.

Another option is to sit in the tub with about three inches of flouride-free hot water and thirty-six ounces of 3% hydrogen peroxide, for ten to fiveteen minutes. While in the tub, change positions so that for a few minutes, all of the different parts of your body are submerged, except your head. And splash the oxygen rich water over your body too.

With either of these methods, you'll probably feel some tingling or stinging, and these are areas with problems in or underneath the skin. As a fair heads up, sometimes the stinging actually hurts a bit and it can last about a half hour. You may also have areas of skin that develop white dots afterward. These dots are signs of a problem in or under the skin and it will stop happening as the problem is removed. And don't worry, the white color will resume to normal, usually within two hours. When the problem is gone, you'll no longer have the burning sensation, or the white spots.

Hydrogen peroxide can be drying too, so use coconut oil daily as a lotion while using it, and I wouldn't recommend doing either of these methods more than twice a week. If your skin is sensitive or becoming dry, dilute your hydrogen peroxide or use it less frequently. After any tingling or sting-ing is gone, you'll can forgo these methods, use them only once a month, or just use them when needed.

Hydrogen peroxide can also lighten your hair a bit, so you'll want to keep it away from your hair and eyebrows. And if it's going to be a problem if some of your body hair is bleached, you might not want to use these methods. For areas like your face and neck, soak some gauze in hydrogen peroxide and rub it on after you've applied some coconut oil. You can also do this for problem areas, like pockets of waste, several times a day for cleansing of targeted areas. Just take breaks when your skin tells you you've had enough.

As a bonus, hydrogen peroxide can remove light wrinkles and make deeper ones less deep—with the effects noticeable relatively quickly. Just use it with coconut oil regularly for lasting results and exfoliate with a washcloth afterward. Also, with either coconut oil or hydrogen peroxide skin cleansing, know that your skin can breakout afterwards, and it's just due to the detoxification going under your skin. So remember, it's temporary—and as with acne in general, it's just your body's way of eliminating toxins.

If you have stubborn problems in the head area that may manifest themselves as thinking problems, concentration problems, migraines, etc., I, personally, would use hydrogen peroxide on my scalp too, after applying coconut oil, and not worry about minor hair color changes, which often take several uses to even be noticeable. The scalp area can be hard to reach with the enemas, yet this reaches it fairly easily. But, you'll need to make your own decisions whether to do this or not. This can be done in the shower and after rubbing it into your scalp for a few minutes, just rinse your hair well.

***For all methods using hydrogen peroxide in this section, use a brand *without* added chemical stabilizers, which are listed in the ingredients as "stabilizers" or as "stabilized" hydrogen peroxide. Aaron Brands® and GoodSense® offer 3% hydrogen peroxide without stabilizers, making them great choices. You can also buy 35% food grade hydrogen peroxide and *carefully* dilute it with twelve times as much water before use. Just read up on this first and use extreme caution with the 35% solution, if you're doing it this way. I, personally, prefer the 3% without the added stabilizers.

Sinus Cleansing

Sinus cleansing is an important step if you have candida in your sinuses—where it commonly lodges once it has left your colon. Since head colds are common, and it's likely that much of the previous debris was never fully eliminated, sinus cleansing can be beneficial even for someone without candida in his or her sinuses. It's also great for other problems above the neck, but it shouldn't be used if you've had ear surgery.

To cleanse your sinuses you'll need a neti pot (which is like a small teapot for nasal cleansing), purified water, and a little sea salt and coconut oil. To do this, warm about a third cup of water and dissolve in a dab of coconut oil and a quarter teaspoon of un-ionized sea salt. Then, making sure it's warm but not hot, add it all to your neti pot. Now, tilt your head to one side and allow the solution to enter the higher nostril, and drain it out the other one, over a sink. When a little is in your nose, you can also inhale quickly through your nose and spit out the debris. Then, just repeat with the other side and continue until you've used all of the solution or until you've had enough. When you're done, blow your nose *and* suck in and spit to remove the debris. Both of these methods are important because they tend to remove problems from different areas.

For more aggressive cleansing that may be needed for sinus infections and chronic problems, you can also use four teaspoons of purified water with one teaspoon 3% hydrogen peroxide in your neti pot. After you've used a little, rub your nose and sinuses firmly to distribute the solution and blow your nose and suck in and spit to remove the debris. Doing this, you may see mucus with a white foam being released. The foam is caused by the hydrogen peroxide killing pathogens and you'll stop seeing it as the problem is removed. Also, know that this can burn, sometimes quite a bit, as it's killing whatever needs to be killed and if this is a problem, dilute your solution even further. However, when the area is free of bacteria, viruses, and candida, it will no longer burn.

Hydrogen peroxide sinus cleansing is best used when there's a problem, but it's not for long-term or consistent use. It can be used three times a day in this manner for problems, but not for more than five days in a row. After five days, it's best to use this only a few times a week, while needed, and use coconut oil and sea salt for more regular use. For sinus problems, you can also do hydrogen peroxide and coconut oil skin cleansing around your face and throat daily too. Candida and filth from these areas can drain into your sinuses and continually re-infect them. When doing this, be sure to massage deeply any areas that you feel tingling or stinging as these are signs of problems.

You should also know that if there's a problem in your sinuses, sometimes it gets worse before it gets better. So, understand that it's just part of the cleansing process as your body is loosening what needs to be removed.

Deep-tissue Massages

Massages are often seen as a luxury item, but when you consider that they break up stagnation and break down pockets of waste, you might begin to see them as more of a necessity than a luxury. Deep tissue massages can help you remove a lot of filth while cleansing and they're also extremely helpful with stubborn knots or lumps that you're having trouble loosening on your own. So, find a good masseuse and have him or her concentrate on your knots to help break up those pockets of waste, so you can remove them. If you can find someone who does a massage technique called "meridian cleansing," try that as well. Either way, do an enema using coffee after your massage to remove the toxins your massage has loosened. If you can manage it, having a deep-tissue massage once a week while cleansing is an excellent plan.

Exercise

Exercise is also extremely helpful while cleansing—as long as you're up for it. Even five minutes of jogging or a half hour walk can help bring blood to areas that it might not regularly reach if you lead a more sedentary lifestyle—and this will allow you to cleanse those areas. Yoga is great too, or even have a dance party around the house to get your blood moving. Aerobic exercise is particularly helpful after any of the retention enemas or while coconut oil mini-fasting—as long as you're not overly tired or experiencing detoxification symptoms.

Juice Fasting

Juice fasting accelerates the cleansing process and encourages very deep cleansing. When your body has no solid food to digest, it can divert more energy to cleansing, so adding a few days of fasting each month to your program can Super-charge your results. If you're up for it, it's highly recommended.

Juice fasting is also an easy way to lose weight quickly and seven days of fasting can easily mean the loss of ten or more pounds for someone who has weight to lose. How many people want to lose ten pounds quickly and easily? However, if you're already thin, you generally won't lose much weight with fasting, possibly only a pound or two in the same time frame. And, if you follow the guidelines below, you won't be hungry and you'll be consuming considerable nutrition through the fresh juices.

So, to juice fast, just cut out solid food and increase your intake of fresh squeezed or blended (and strained) juices and psyllium drinks (without baking soda). You'll want to take in three or four psyllium drinks each day which will keep you full, and then have as many fresh-squeezed or blended juices as you desire. Ideally, this would four or more large juices each day, and ideally with lots of green juices. (Appendix C)

You can fast for up to a week on this program, or just on weekends, if it's easier for you. But before you do either, prepare your body by doing *The Cleaning Up! Cleanse* for at least two weeks first so you don't induce detoxification that your body is unable to handle. You'll also want to do the enemas daily while fasting.

In addition, it's important to end your fast carefully, particularly if you are fasting longer than a day or two. To end your fast, you'll bring solid food back in *slowly*, and in the order below—to allow your digestive system time to wake up peacefully.

The proper order for reintroducing foods is fresh fruit or blended vegetables first, then raw vegetables, then cooked vegetables, then carbohydrates, and then protein. Introduce one of these each day, and be careful with your diet approximately the same number of days you've fasted.

Fasting allows every cell of your body to cleanse deeply, but please respect the importance of ending a fast properly. Not doing so can damage your digestive tract, particularly if you eat too much or introduce complex foods too soon, especially with longer fasts. People have been hospitalized as a result of ending a fast improperly, so it's really not something to take lightly.

Those with Type 1 diabetes, hypoglycemia, wasting diseases, or serious liver or kidney impairment shouldn't fast. It's also best not to take medication while fasting, so use caution if you are on medication. It may not be appropriate to exercise aerobically while fasting, so take it easy if needed. Be sure and rest as needed, too.

Coconut Oil Mini-Fasting

For extremely powerful candida cleansing and detoxification, you can also add in mini-fasting using lots of coconut oil. Because coconut oil is such a powerful anti-bacterial, anti-fungal, anti-viral and anti-cancer substance, it's great for many other problems in the body too. Actually, combined with the standard methods in this cleanse, this is one of the most powerful methods in this book for breaking up solid lumps quickly. To boot, it's a delicious and filling soup.

Just blend it all with a cup of hot or warm water.

* ✳ 2-3 tomatoes
* ✳ Juice of one lemon or two limes
* ✳ 2 to 4 cloves of garlic
* ✳ 8 tablespoons of coconut oil
* ✳ Sea salt to taste

To mini-fast using coconut oil, just make this coconut oil soup two or three of your meals each day. In this manner, you can easily take in sixteen plus tablespoons of coconut oil a day—which will make for some of the most aggressive cleansing you can do. However, because this is so powerful, it's best to have cleansed *at least* six weeks before adding it in. Even with some deep cleansing first, it's likely that most people will experience detoxification symptoms, so do this when you can be around the house to rest. And know that your detoxification symptoms will lessen, and then disappear, as you become cleaner.

Coconut oil mini-fasting can be done one or two days a week while cleansing, so it can be done on weekends. Or, if you can find a few weeks to do it daily, it makes for powerful and intense detoxification—even with stubborn problems. The only real risk you run by doing it aggressively is burning out on coconut oil and having the flavor turn on you as described in Chapter 10, in which case, you'll need to stop. But, it's easy to have this soup for breakfast and lunch and then enjoy another dinner. Or have the soup for dinner too. If you want to slow it down, just use a little less oil. And if possible, do your enemas in the morning to allow the oil to remain in your body overnight.

Remember, having the psyllium drinks after lots of coconut oil may cause some cramping, but it'll really clean out your small intestine. But, if this sounds like too much, just skip the psyllium drinks when you're doing this. You can also multiply the intestinal cleansing effect by having a cup or two of senna tea each day while you're doing coconut oil mini-fasting and the psyllium drinks—and know that you'll be using the rest room very regularly. When you doing coconut oil mini-fasting, you'll also want to hold off on the retention enemas—because chances are decent that you won't be able to retain them long enough for them to do their work.

For major candida problems and almost *any* other serious problem in the body (including cancer, AIDS, dementia, etc.), I'd add this in *regularly*, with regular cleansing, but only *after* I'd done some deep and aggressive cleansing first. With dementia and other brain problems, we're lucky because coconut oil can cross the blood brain barrier to do its work.

Coconut oil mini-fasting is also a great way to reduce the total time needed for thorough cleansing and address other stubborn problems, even without major diagnosed issues.

For variety, you can use any of the tomato, avocado, or broccoli soups in Appendix B, as well. Just use the recipes with eight tablespoons of coconut oil. If you'd like your meals to be a little more substantial, you can also pour your soups over a bowl of chopped veggies.

More Coconut Oil

For general cleansing and female gynecological problems, including yeast infections, bladder infections, endometriosis, or sexually transmitted diseases, coconut oil can be used internally too. Just insert a tablespoon and lie down on a towel with your hips raised for ten minutes each day. Then, flip over and lie on your stomach for further distribution. Females can also douche twice a week with a 1:1 3% hydrogen peroxide and water solution—or daily with two teaspoons of baking soda in a cup of water. It's best to do either in a bathtub, while warm from a shower. It's also best to do this on your knees, with your head to the ground, and with a rear insertion, for best distribution and so you can retain some of it for a minute. Then, discontinue when it's no longer needed. For serious problems, start slower with hydrogen peroxide and work up because it may burn.

Men can also use coconut oil and hydrogen peroxide topically for many sexually transmitted diseases. For men and women, a 2:1 mixture of coconut oil and baking soda can be used topically too. Just apply it after bathing, rub it in a few minutes and wash it off. Then, use coconut oil over your whole body, before dressing. For problems of this sort, deeply massage your abdomen while doing the enemas too.

Red Beets

Red beets are powerful blood cleansers and they're known to break up cancers and tumors quickly. In fact, a Hungarian oncologist in the 50s, Dr. Ferenczi, was eliminating tumors in his patients by having them drink large amounts of beet juice daily. Beets are powerful because they boost our phase II detoxification enzymes and these enzymes help us remove many man-made chemicals. At the same time, red beets also repair our DNA and since many common chemicals and lifestyle habits damage our DNA, DNA repair is more needed than you might think.

Beets can be added to your program as foods, juices and in the enemas, but only after the large majority of candida has been cleared from your blood. To clear the large majority of candida from your blood often takes at least a couple of months, but it can take longer, so you'll need to judge by what you see coming out of you. (What candida looks like, p. 115) Basically, anything white is candida, but it can have a yellowish or brownish tinge if it's older. You'll wait before adding beets in because even though beets are antifungal, they also contain some sugar. However, when you're ready, you can start using beets in your enemas, using the beet recipes in Appendix B, and/or drinking the juice of one or two red beets a day.

Gallbladder Cleanse

This process cleans the gallbladder and painlessly removes gall-stones. It's been around for ages and I've done it several times over the years. In all, I've released approximately two dozen marble-sized gallstones, a hundred pea-sized stones, and thousands of sand-like mini-stones. I also believe that just every adult has gallstones, whether they know it or not. Gallbladder cleansing is also great for insomnia or other sleep issues. Actually, it eliminated my three-year struggle with insomnia—overnight. Plus, it's helpful for allergies and upper back and shoulder tightness. But, for this to be effective, please note that you'll need to be precise with the timing.

So, here are the protocols:

✱ Have a no-fat breakfast and lunch (no oils, nuts, etc.), and don't eat after two in the afternoon. By staying away from fat, it allows pressure to built in your liver which makes the stones easier to remove. By not eating after two, it helps ensure you won't feel sick later on. If you're using coconut oil in the enemas, foods, or as a skin lotion, avoid doing so for three days before embarking on this process.

✱ At 6 pm: Drink two tablespoons of Epsom salts dissolved in sixteen ounces of purified water to open your bile ducts so the stones can pass through painlessly. For your Epsom salts, be sure to use magnesium sulfate, and not magnesium sulfate heptahydrate, as the later can cause some burning upon exiting the body.

✻ At 8 pm: Drink the Epsom salts mixture again.

✻ At 9:45 pm: Stir the juice of two or three lemons into a half cup of light olive oil. Then, go to the bathroom and get ready for bed.

✻ At 10 pm on the dot: Stir and drink the lemon juice and olive oil mixture. Drink it while standing up, and as quickly as possible. Try to finish it all in five minutes or less and then *immediately* lie down in bed. Lie on your right side with your knees pulled up to your chest and don't move for twenty minutes. The first twenty minutes of stillness are critical to getting the stones out. Then, just stay still until you fall asleep. The olive oil will cause your gallbladder to expand and contract, which pushes the stones into your colon for removal.

✻ First thing in the morning, but not before 6 am: Have another Epsom salts drink.

✻ Two hours later: Drink the Epsom salts mixture one last time, and expect to use the restroom shortly afterward. You'll see the stones come out in your release. They can be different colors, but are often green, as they are coated with bile. You'll see them easily, as the cholesterol in the center of each stone makes them float.

You may feel nauseous the next day, so do this when you can rest the day after if needed. While it's not common, it's also not unheard of to wake up in the middle of the night and vomit after doing this. If this happens, it's because you've stirred up more toxins in your gallbladder than your body could handle, and your body wanted them out—quickly.

So, it's nothing to be concerned about, but it means that your gallbladder was pretty toxic. You'll also want to have cleansed for several weeks prior to doing this to ensure your bowel is clean to allow the stones to pass through and to help make sure you feel better during the process. This can be done every six weeks until all of your stones are removed.

Mouth Cleansing

Oxygen-rich hydrogen peroxide can also be used to cleanse the mouth and kill candida in the tongue, where it often gets a foothold and can be hard to reach with other methods. As a bonus, hydrogen peroxide also mildly bleaches stains from our teeth. So, just use a capful of 3% hydrogen peroxide diluted with two or three times as much water, and brush your teeth and tongue with it. This can be done once a week and more often for problems like thrush. You can also gargle with a 3:1 solution of water to hydrogen peroxide, which is great for conquering sore throats.

Balancing Hormones Naturally

Many hormonal problems are due to toxicity in the body—particularly an abundance of environmental estrogens, which are chemicals that mimic our natural hormones. As such, deep cleansing helps considerably with hormonal problems. However, maca root is also a powerful balancer of hormones. Maca root nourishes our glands and acts as an adaptagen—meaning it works to balance our hormones however the body needs them to be balanced. It's also well known to increase sex drive and function, particularly in men.

Just a teaspoon of maca root daily is helpful to help balance hormones and often works wonders for PMS and problems during menopause. As a note, there are several varieties of maca and some taste sweet, while others are bitter. So, if you're having trouble with the flavor, try a different supplier, as you might be using a more bitter variety. You can also add maca to banana smoothies, with stevia, to improve the flavor.

The Asian herb dong quai can also be beneficial for balancing hormones, giving energy and boosting the immune system. Look for it as a root and seep it in boiled water for about ten minutes to make a tea. You can use a teaspoon per cup and add peppermint tea for flavor, and stevia to sweeten. Then, enjoy regularly. However, avoid dong quai if you are pregnant.

Chakra Clearing

As we talked about, at times while cleansing you may experience negative energy as a cleansing release, and you may just experience it in the course of your life. Sometimes, it can be hard to let go of, so let's talk about some ways to clear negative energy, so it doesn't get the best of you.

This method and the next two are to help you clear negative energy whenever it's needed, and personally, I find chakra clearing to be the most powerful of the three. So, to clear negative energy from your chakras, or energy centers, first you'll need to be aware of where your chakras are and what energy runs through them. So, let's start there.

We actually have seven energy points, or chakras, that run down the center of our bodies and each is connected with different energies. I'll list the chakras and their corresponding energies, and if you think you might have repressed or stuck energy in any of these areas, this method can help you clear them out.

Your first chakra is at the base of your spine and it's connected to grounding, stability, and security. If you're feeling insecure or afraid in a survival type way, this energy is being affected.

Your second chakra is just below your belly button and it's connected to emotions, sexuality, and intimacy. If you have uncontrolled or repressed emotions, are over or under sexualized, or have intimacy issues, this is the area you'll want to work on. Some of the male sexual energy is also in the first chakra.

Your third chakra is just below the bottom of your rib cage and it's your center for vitality, desire, and power. If you're feeling weak, lethargic, or powerless, this is the area you'll want to address.

Your fourth chakra is in your chest, at the height of your heart, and is related to hope, compassion, loving yourself and loving others. If you find yourself not loving yourself or others, or are having a hard time letting go of a wrong done to you, your heart chakra is probably in need of some clearing. Other good times to clear your heart chakra are if you're feeling indecisive, afraid of getting hurt, or sorry for yourself.

Your fifth chakra is in your throat and it's all about creativity and good communication skills. If you're not speaking your truth with poise or standing up for yourself, this is the area you'll want to address.

Your sixth chakra is in your forehead and it's linked to clairvoyance, psychic abilities, and intuition.

Your seventh chakra is at the top of your head and it's linked to cosmic consciousness and the ability to achieve enlightenment. It should be noted that it's possible for most every human to achieve enlightenment.

For visuals of where the chakras are located, just do a search on the Internet. Then, to clear energy from your chakras, hold a tablespoon of sea salt in the palm of a closed hand and lay down and put that hand over the chakra you want to work on. Just hold the salt there for about ten minutes and let the energy clear on its own. You can also hold the salt over cancers, lumps you're breaking up, your shoulders, or other areas of tension in your body to remove negative energy from these points too. Chunky sea salt is more effective than fine grained, but either will work. Just use fresh sea salt every few times you do this and obviously, don't consume the salt afterward.

You should also know that with energy clearing, sometimes it will be an almost instantaneous process as the salt pulls the energy away and it's gone forever. However, if it's a deeply rooted issue or there is a bunch of toxicity in the area too, it can be a longer process and can require that the toxicity be removed for the energy to clear completely. As we've talked about, stuck energy and toxicity often go hand in hand.

Cleansing Breathwork

Another way to clear negative energy is simply to breath in and out deeply through your mouth repeatedly, and also occasionally hold your breath for a few seconds at the top and bottom of each breath. This helps push out the old energy—and often you'll feel the palms of your hands warm as the energy is exiting. It's also great for a regular breathwork too and it tends to promote spiritual connectedness.

Hot and Cold Showers

The final energy clearing technique is just to take cold showers, as cold water absorbs negative energy. While in the shower, you can also literally wipe the energy from the top of your head, your back and shoulders by brushing with your hands the areas just outside your body, where energy resides. While the effects can be instantaneous, this may need to be done repeatedly for lasting results.

You can also alternative between hot and cold water in the shower, for comfort and a little more detoxification power too. The gist of alternating hot and cold showers is to make them as hot and as cold as you can stand, and spend a few minutes in each while alternating between them. By alternating between hot and cold water, it forces your muscles and cells to expand and contract which aids in detoxification.

Developing Love-Based Thinking

Just as important as knowing how to clear negative energy, is knowing how to avoid creating it in the first place. A lot of this starts in the mind and it has a lot to do with how we process information and events in our lives. It also starts with the knowledge that there are two fundamental energy and emotional sources: love and fear. And when we live in a state of love, we'll have a totally different life experience than if we live in a state of fear.

Love-based thinking also tends to become more natural, and simply how we think, once we've cleansed deeply and are eating nature's foods, especially raw foods, but it can be consciously practiced too.

So, the easiest way to jump into love-based thinking (and out of fear-based thinking) is to simply live in the present and accept everything that comes in your life. Living in the present means keeping your thoughts out of either the past or the future, and beginning to recognize all of the gifts and guidance the Universe is giving you in the present (which we'll often miss if our minds are occupied with either the future or the past). It's also about recognizing that we do have power in our lives and that we can refuse what we don't want while creating what we do. In fact, in a lot of ways, love-based thinking is about giving up control and any need to control, while assuming our power and letting the Universe be our guide.

To get started on this path, one of the most powerful things you can do is to begin accepting situations that might otherwise cause you anger, judgement, worry or other fear-based emotions. And the words to do this are simply, "It is what it is." So, if you find yourself in any fear-based emotion, simply stop and accept the situation for what it is. Say and truly mean, "It is what it is." When you've done so, you'll often find a better way to handle it simply comes to you. Or perhaps you'll see that the "bad," really wasn't bad after all. In fact, many seemlying "bad" situations are often the Universe's way of providing a gift, that you may not recognize until later. However, if you don't process the situation in a love-based state, you might miss the gift and also create more drama in your life by your fear-based reaction.

Love-based thinking also about looking at your thoughts and decisions and determining if they are coming from a place of love, or a place of fear. If they're coming from a place of fear, I'd suggest that a better solution is out there, for whatever situation you're working on. This applies not only to major life decisions, but to small everyday ones as well. Actually, the little everyday ones build our larger ones, so in many ways they are very important.

If you're stuck in a fear-based place, and we've all been there, the easiest way out of it is to start being grateful for all the good things that you do have—even if just for the air you have to breath. In a state of gratitude, you'll be energetically receptive to more good things, than from a place of fear, so it's a way to call good things into your life.

From here, you'll simply want to begin trusting yourself and your emotions which will often give you clues to your highest path. You'll also want to start trusting in the synchronicities that will likely appear in your life. Synchronicitous events are often the Universe's ways of guiding you, so it's important to see them for what they are. Most people will have a grand old time if they just follow Universal guidance, while maintaining a present centered, love-based state, and, of course, the more people living this way, the better it becomes for everyone.

Natural Birth Control

You probably know that I'm not a fan of putting any chemicals in or on the body and some more chemicals that can be eliminated are birth control pills or other chemically oriented birth control methods. However, to practice natural birth control is a little different than is commonly known—and the responsibility actually lies with the male. So, how is it done?

Well, it turns out that sperm don't like heat and by bathing, or simply submerging the testes, in 116 degrees water, which thankfully is just *below* the pain threshold, for forty-five minutes a day for twenty-one days, a male becomes reliably sterile for the next six months. Doing this in 110 degree water, which isn't even all *that* hot, for twenty-one days produces sterility for the next four months—and it's just repeated when the allotted time is up, until a child is desired. You'll also need to add more hot water during the process to keep it hot enough.

This method dates back to the time of Hippocrates and it's been shown to be completely effective over a ten year period with a group of males in India, who were also easily able to have children when they stopped. It works because sperm needs to be several degrees cooler than body temperature—which is actually why it hangs outside the body. In fact, sperm cell death happens at 95 degrees, while normal cell death happens at 108 degrees—so this effectively kills sperm for a limited but extended period of time—and all without chemicals or hormone alteration.

Dry Skin Brushing

Skin brushing is an easy method that helps your skin breath by removing your top layers of skin. Essentially, it opens your pores and allows your body purge its toxins through your skin, while stimulating your lymphatic system to purge its toxins too. The lymphatic system is fluid system in your body that feeds your cells and removes cellular waste, just as your blood does. However, unlike your blood, which has your heart as a pump, the lymphatic system needs to be simulated to move. This is generally done through exercise, but skin brushing also helps move it along.

Dry skin brushing involves brushing your skin, similarly to how you'd brush your hair. It starts with dry skin and a soft, dry, natural bristled brush . Then, starting at your feet, begin brushing your skin, using strokes toward your heart. Move up your legs and do your back and stomach too. Finally, brush your arms and upper body, with each stroke toward your heart. It's easy to do in the shower, before bathing, and afterward your dead skin will head down the drain.

In doing this, you'll want to brush hard enough so that your skin turns a little red, but not hard enough to cause pain or irritation. Be sure and also be gentle with thin skin and avoid brushing areas with rashes or broken skin. Just brush for a few minutes a day and within a few weeks it's likely you'll notice a big improvement in your skin.

Quitting Smoking

Detoxifying your body can be an easy way to quit smoking and drop other chemically addictive behaviors, because you'll be removing the chemicals in your body that are *causing* your cravings. To cleanse to quit, start consuming five to ten large, fresh-squeezed fruit or vegetable juices each day and adopt a mostly raw fruit and vegetable diet. Enjoy your favorite juices and don't worry about consuming fruit, even with a candida problem. At this point, it's more important to conquer your cravings.

Start your day with a large juice and have more throughout the day. It's critical that you have a large juice whenever the addictive urge arises—as flooding your body with fresh juice can instantly wipe out the cravings. And if the craving is gone after your juice—just don't have that cigarette. The herb lobelia also calms cravings, and you can start using it a few weeks before beginning the aggressive juicing.

It's important that you're near your juicer during this process, so begin on a weekend. You may also be tired and want to rest. Using enemas also helps pull those chemicals out of your body and will make the entire process faster and easier.

If you have a cigarette or two during the process, don't worry —just keep going. Generally, the cravings will cease within a few days and by the end of the week, you'll simply need to manage your behavior—and that's far easier than managing behavior that's tied to addictive cravings.

Wiping Out Ear Infections

Ear infections are often caused by a virus, bacteria, or fungus in the ear and an easy way to get rid of them is to use the diluted juice of garlic in your ear.

Just blend two cloves of garlic with a third cup of water, and strain the mixture so you're only using the liquid. Then, tilt your head to the side and pour the liquid into your ear. Hold it in for a minute before tilting your head to the other side to drain it out and then just rinse your ear in your next shower.

Know that this may be painful as the garlic is killing the virus, bacteria, or fungus, so if you have a low tolerance for pain, use more water. When the problem is gone, the pain will be too.

Getting Rid of Athlete's Foot

If you have athlete's foot, open a probiotic capsule and sprinkle some over the infected area. Then, add the rest to some cotton socks and wear them during the day. Repeat before bed and do this daily until the problem is gone. Hydrogen peroxide skin cleansing, when done on the feet, can wipe out athlete's foot too.

Regrowing Teeth and Bone

Most people don't know it, but our teeth can regrow themselves which is especially helpful if you have a cavity and want to avoid fillings. I've regrown several of my own teeth, and it's easy to do, but it requires consistency and patience. Actually, it requires a little more consistency than I sometimes have for it, so I'm still working on a couple too.

In any case, to regrow your teeth, you'll need plenty of minerals in your body, and for this, we get those minerals from eggshells. Consuming eggshells also helps build bone and has even been shown to reverse osteoporosis too. Eggshells contain 27 minerals and they're very similar in make up to our own teeth and bone, so they give us the materials needed for the work. We'll also use comfrey leaf which is an herb that encourages the rapid regrowth of cells.

So, just get a couple cartons of organic eggs, crack and clean the shells, and soak the shells in boiling water for a minute to kill any pathogens. Then, let them dry in the sun. When they're dry, grind your shells in a coffee grinder until they're powdered and store them covered and refrigerated. Now, you'll want to eat a ½ to 1 teaspoon of ground shells each day until the work is done. You can take them with a spoon and wash them down with water or you can add your shells to banana-based smoothies, but be sure to drink the shells that sink to the bottom too. If you're doing a teaspoon of shells, have a ½ teaspoon, twice a day.

To regrow and build your bones, you'll need to consume the eggshells regularly. To regrow your teeth, you'll also want to bring the comfrey in contact with your teeth and gums. So, start by rehydrating a tablespoon or so of dried comfrey leaf by letting it soak in water for a half hour to an hour. Then, just pack the wet leaves along your gums and let them sit for an hour or longer each day. For the fastest regrowth possible, you can also sleep with the comfrey along your gumlines. After you're done, just spit it out and for children, reduce the eggshells and comfrey by half, or more. You'll also want to drink a few cups comfrey leaf tea daily, so just seep a couple tablespoons of the leaves in three cups of hot water for ten minutes to make a tea, then sweeten with stevia. You can also swish the tea between your teeth and consume the leaves in your tea.

To regrow your teeth, it can take a few months of daily use and sometimes it takes longer. It'll take longer if you have multiple teeth to regrow, if the holes are large, or if your bones need rebuilding too, because your body may prioritize rebuilding your bones before your teeth. In any case, as a preventative measure, you can also eat the shells and drink comfrey leaf tea a few times a month too. Personally I think it's a great idea because fossil records show that today's humans have very holey bones compared to our long ago ancestors.

Comfrey also has a dark tea-like color, so brush your teeth with baking soda and hydrogen peroxide after packing it along your gumlines to prevent staining. This may regrow teeth with veneers on them a little, but it generally won't push fillings out of your teeth. As a caution though, if you haven't gotten MSG out of your diet—and it's in all types of processed foods—I wouldn't recommend this much calcium; it can exacerbate the toxic effects of MSG. Greens, particularly green drinks, are another mineral-rich source and they can be substituted for the eggshells if desired, although it may not be as fast.

Chapter 13

Ongoing Eating— Easy Tips for a Big Difference!

Many people will want to upgrade their long-term dietary plan after cleansing and since meat and junk food cravings commonly disappear with cleansing, it's an optimal time to do it.

So, remember: healthy eating starts in the grocery store. Purchasing organic ensures that your food tastes better— and that it doesn't contain toxic residue. Buying more fresh fruits, veggies, seeds, and nuts and eliminating processed foods, sugary foods, and animal products will be a gigantic step forward for most people. These simple steps will also dramatically reduce the number of chemicals you'll be putting in your body each day, and your body will thank you today and in the years to come. So, here are some easy tips to get you started.

✱ Make two or more of your meals each day from fresh, unheated fruits and vegetables. To make this easy, simply continue eating your favorite salads, vegetable wraps, and blended soups regularly. You'll also want to add fresh fruit once your candida issues are under control, which can be a wonderful breakfast.

✱ Enjoy raw, soaked nuts and seeds regularly for protein, healthy fat and as a key source of tryptophan to promote healthy moods. Most seeds and nuts should be soaked in purified probiotic water before they are eaten. This makes them easier to digest, activates naturally occurring enzymes, and helps remove some of the mold that's often on them.

✱ Keep a variety of raw mushrooms in your diet, and move beyond the standard button mushrooms too. I think two to four cups of raw mushrooms a week is a good game plan for most people. Mushrooms also keep you full, so they're great carbohydrate replacements. I use mushrooms regularly in salads, veggie wraps, and as a "bread" for my nut pates. Many are delicious topped with sea salt and fresh herbs too. It's also important to know that mushrooms are best fresh and they don't last long, so eat them quickly. If they've turned even slightly slimy, toss them as they become a little toxic at this stage. If you're doing white button mushrooms, you'll also want to check to make sure they haven't been irradiated. Shiitake mushrooms are best with white, as opposed to yellow gills, underneath.

✱ Keep the green drinks in your diet, and especially if you're following a vegetarian or vegan diet, enjoy grass drinks regularly to stock up on the cancer busting, strength promoting

CLA. The grass drinks are another way to bring forward your spiritual connectedness, especially if you use them, and raw nuts, as replacements for animal eating.

✱ Enjoy a cup or two of raw, unpasteurized sauerkraut each week to keep your gut loaded with protective healthy bacteria. These healthy bacteria also produce B12 in your body.

✱ Have pineapple and papaya regularly to stock up on digestive enzymes, but make sure your papaya is organic or not from Hawaii to avoid the genetically modified varieties.

✱ Enjoy raw cabbage, beets, cilantro, and seaweed regularly to benefit from their ability to remove chemicals and heavy metals from the body.

✱ Use coconut oil abundantly and if you're cooking, use it as your primary cooking oil. In addition to having tremendous health benefits, coconut oil is the only oil that can stand the heat of cooking without creating free radicals. Coconut oil works wonderfully for cooking, in most recipes, and in some salad dressings. It's also a delicious "butter" on popcorn, potatoes, rice, or bread.

✱ Use unrefined sea salt instead of table salt. Unlike nutrient-stripped table salt, sea salt is full of minerals and has the ability to break down in the body. Grey or pink salts have more nutrients than white sea salt.

✱ Drink extra purified water. Water keeps your tissues hydrated, flushes toxins from your body, and encourages bowel movements. On colder days, you may prefer to drink your water warm. Either way, make sure your water is purified, as tap water contains chlorine and often fluoride, among other poisons. If your city fluorinates, be sure you're purifying with either reverse osmosis, a distiller, or an activated alumina filter to remove most or all of the fluoride.

* Drink herbal teas and try some powerful ones like cat's claw or dandelion root. Sweeten them with organic honey or agave (if you don't have candida) or stevia (if you do). These are great replacement beverages for regular coffee drinkers.

* Buy organic whenever possible. Most people think that pesticides are solely found on the exterior of their foods. However, with rain, pesticides are drawn into the soil and they become part of the "food" for the plant—and then part of the entire plant. Similarly, they become part of you when you consume them, as neither plants nor humans have the ability to effectively remove pesticides. Since pesticides are designed to kill living organisms, using them in our food seems a touch insane. But organic is about more than pesticides. Radiation is also used on non-organic vegetables—and the notion that this is safe is laughable.

* Say goodbye to your microwave. Microwaves are known to turn healthy food into carcinogens while destroying most of the nutrition in food. Why even keep one in the house?

* Avoid GMO (genetically modified) foods like the plague. This means avoiding all non-organic corn, corn products (like chips, tortillas, corn syrup), soy, soy products (including tofu), lecithin (derived from soy), white sugar (from sugar beets), products with white sugar in them, Hawaiian papaya, cottonseed oil, canola, canola oil, and margarine (de-

rived from canola oil). Seventy percent of all of the processed foods found in traditional grocery stores contain GMOs. With no labeling requirements these days, it's a fairly dangerous game of buyer beware.[9] Perhaps you want to choose a grocery store that is committed to keeping GMOs off the shelves and just avoid processed foods altogether? Farm animals are regularly fed genetically modified soy and corn too, so to avoid consuming GMOs secondhand you'll need organic meat, eggs, and dairy, if you eat these substances.

✻ Avoid sugar as much as possible, including hidden sugars: sucrose, glucose, fructose, maltose, corn syrup, etc. Use stevia if you enjoy it. Those without candida or sugar issues can use agave, dates, raw organic honey, or grade-B maple syrup to sweeten. Stevia has no sugar, and agave, dates, honey and maple syrup have a high sugar, but they are also healthful. However, even natural sweeteners like honey, dates, agave, and maple syrup should also be used in moderation. Honey should be organic due to the possibility GMO contamination and if your honey isn't organic, it's best to use agave instead.

✻ Avoid white rice, pasta, and white flour, as they're all stripped of their nutritional value from bleaching and refinement. Actually, the work they require from your body to remove them generally cancels out any nutritional benefits. You might also want to leave whole wheat, barley, and rye products out of your diet, due to the number of people who

---

9   For more on GMOs, their health hazards, and the cover-up of these dangers, read *Seeds of Deception* by Jeffrey Smith. For current information about GMO foods, visit www.responsibletechnology.org.

have unrecognized gluten intolerance issues. Better alternatives are brown rice, sprouted grain, and whole grain products. Boiled and baked potatoes are also good replacements for pasta and other flour products.

✷ Avoid chemical sweeteners, especially aspartame. With all of the detrimental effects they're known have on health, the fact that many chemical sweeteners are still legally allowed in our food supply is amazing. Aspartame, believe it or not, was once listed as a chemical warfare agent. However, because of consumer rejection of aspartame, it's being renamed; the new name is AminoSweet®.

✷ Eliminate or keep processed foods to a minimum. Processed foods add little nutritional value, and many require so much effort on the part of your body to remove them that the effort outweighs any nutritional value they might offer. Most are also packed with chemicals and contain GMOs.

✷ Eliminate fast food, junk food, and sodas. These are all acid-forming in the body, chemical intensive, and polluting, all of which is strongly correlated with disease. In addition, they provide no nutritional value. Many processed foods and fast foods also contain MSG, which is a seriously toxic substance. MSG goes by lots of names, and it's common in ingredients with the words "protein," "hydrolyzed," "yeast," or "glutamate."

✷ Eliminate or drink alcohol in moderation. Its hazardous effects on the liver are well-known. You'll also want keep coffee to a minimum too, or give it up altogether. Herbal teas are great replacements.

A Note about Heart Health

Cayenne pepper is wonderful for the heart and has been known to stop a heart attack instantly. Cayenne pepper improves circulation and is a wonderful addition to the daily routine of anyone with heart troubles. In my opinion, a quarter teaspoon of cayenne pepper each day is a must for anyone with heart troubles, along with a vegetarian diet and a clean, probiotic-infused colon. If you have heart trouble, you may want to try this for a few months and see if your doctor notices a difference. Many will notice a significant improvement. For regular consumption, the cinnamon and spice tea on p. 214 can be a delicious way to take it and cayenne can deliciously added to many other teas too. Cayenne is also wonderful in soups, bean and lentil dishes, and vegetable sautés.

❋ Eliminate or keep dairy products to a minimum. Dairy products are mucus-forming and cause a lot of congestion in the body. Usable calcium is more available in green leafy vegetables, so it's better to get your calcium there. The sweet green drinks (Appendix C) are excellent calcium-rich alternatives and if you're going to do dairy, raw dairy is much preferable to pasteurized.

❋ Eliminate or keep animal consumption to a minimum. Animal "products" create a lot of acid waste in the body, and their production wastes natural resources and promotes cruelty and fear, which energetically is passed onto the people consuming the animals. The hormones, antibiotics and other drugs used in "production" are passed on too, and eating lots of animals is strongly correlated with heart disease, the #1 killer in the U.S. So, use only organic, antibiotic-free, free-range meats if you eat meat. In addition, you should know that the human body's protein requirements are met by *one* serving of meat each week. Consuming fish is better than consuming land or air animals because it's easier for the body to break down—but make sure your fish isn't farm-raised or from the Gulf of Mexico. And with all of the fish washing up dead all over the world these days, I personally would give some serious thought to consuming fish at all. In any case, eating more than two servings of animals a week will cause problems over time because the human body really isn't designed to break down animal flesh as food. If we were, we'd have a short digestive tract and high levels of hydrochloric acid in our stomachs. Every animal in nature that consumes other animals has both—yet humans have neither.

✶ Beans and lentils are great replacements for much of the protein that meat eaters derive from the animal kingdom. Just six or seven cups of beans or lentils weekly meets the protein requirements of human beings, and they are easy to prepare and inexpensive.

✶ It's also important to eat proteins and carbohydrates at separate meals. Proteins and carbohydrates require separate and competing enzymes to break them down and when you

eat proteins and carbohydrates together (like meat and potatoes, meat and rice, or meat and bread), your body releases
both sets of enzymes. They essentially cancel each other out,
which hampers digestion and nutrient absorption.

✴ With any foods, it's important to chew them well to aid in
digestion. Also remember that your teeth are in your mouth,
not your stomach.

✴ And finally, be gentle with yourself when making dietary changes and make improvements in stages, if that is
more comfortable for you, instead of making dramatic shifts
overnight. It's not important that you're 100% perfect with
your diet *all* of the time, and you don't need a completely
non-flexible diet. For most people, it's enough to have a very
healthy diet the *large* majority of the time, avoid the really
bad choices consistently, and not worry about the rest. However, those ridding themselves of candida problems will need
to be more stringent until the problem is behind them.

This chapter offers easy tips that are designed to be doable for anyone who wants to make the effort to upgrade
their diet from standard meat, refined carbohydrate and
processed foods diets. However, if you're interested in really taking your energetic vibration to the next level, you can
even trim down this list a bit.

To do this, just keep all, or most all, of your foods directly
from nature—raw or uncooked—unprocessed, and non-
animal derived. An ideal diet would be plenty of salads, raw
soups, raw vegetable wraps, sea vegetables, soaked nuts and

seeds, nut milks, nut pates, nut cereals, sauerkraut, fruit smoothies, nut smoothies, sprouts, a variety of raw mushrooms, coconut oil, green drinks, wild grass drinks, fresh juices, fruit, fresh herbs and herb teas. More complicated raw foods, like raw pizza or cheesecake, are great for treats, but nature really intended us to be eating raw foods a little closer to their natural form.

Many raw foodists also get into dehydrated foods, but the energy really comes from raw *living* foods. So, it's best to use dehydrated foods somewhat sparingly, because even though they are raw, they're also dormant.

I also believe that with this kind of diet, occasional, reasonably healthy diversions are just fine. For a lot of people, I think this is important to remember because it's really about living in a high energy state, and not about having a one hundred percent "perfect" diet all the time. Actually, this type of diet is just a path to bring you to the high energy and spiritual connectedness. In addition, I think that the fear of all or nothing keeps a lot of people from taking this path, so while all is great, it's definitely not required for participation.

Chapter 14

Staying Clean! Reducing Daily Exposure

Now that you're taking the time and effort to clean up your body, you may also want to follow these simple steps to avoid unnecessary toxic exposure. Often times, it's as simple as just picking up different products.

✷ Use coconut oil as your daily skin lotion. It has softening and sunscreen properties, and none of the chemicals found in lotion or sunscreen. Because 90 percent of what you put on your skin makes it into your bloodstream, the more chemicals you can eliminate from your routine, the better.

✷ Use deodorant without aluminum—or cleanse to the point that deodorant is no longer needed. Standard deodorants contain aluminum, which is strongly correlated with Alzheimer's disease and other memory disorders, so aluminum is the last thing you want to be putting on your skin each day. Of course, you'll also want to avoid sodas or other foods packaged in aluminum to further reduce your exposure to the harmful substance.

❋ If you have mercury fillings (called silver fillings) in your mouth, visit a biological dentist and have them replaced. Porcelain is the best choice for replacement and be sure to cleanse using cilantro and coffee enemas after you've had them removed to clean out any metals released during the removal process. If you can make it to Tijuana without being radiated or molested at the airport, they do the removals there at about a tenth the price as in the U.S. Mercury, along with untold other toxic substances, is also in vaccines, and it's best to pass on those as well.

❋ Use toothpaste without fluoride. I know, this contradicts what many have been taught, but as I mentioned, fluoride is the sole ingredient in many rat poisons. Jason® has some great toothpastes and as an alternative, you can use a little coconut oil and baking soda instead.

❋ Use shampoos, conditioners, and body soaps that are light on chemicals. Dr. Bronner's offers a wonderful face and body soap, while Kiss My Face® and Beauty Without Cruelty brands offer good shampoos and conditioners. You can also start washing your hair only every few days, and just rinsing it on off days, if desired. Our hair actually creates more oil as a response to daily washing and it will produce less if you wash it less frequently.

❋ Buy make-up and personal care supplies at trusted health food stores. The products have been prescreened, so it's easy to be safe without having to learn a lot. However, some products with either propyl alcohol or sodium lauryl sulfate (SLS) make it into health food stores, and they should be avoided. Propyl alcohol goes by lots of names, so avoid products with any "prop" in the ingredients. It's common in many products, including antifreeze—in which it's the main ingredient! It's really best to go as light as possible on personal care products and cut out as many as possible from your daily routine. The Environmental Working Group offers a great resource to guide you through the toxicity of personal care items at www.cosmeticsdatabase.com.

✳ Use non-toxic, environmentally friendly cleaning supplies in your home which are often found at health food stores. It's particularly important to use safe cleaning supplies to wash your clothes, in your kitchen, in your bath and on floors that you walk on barefoot. Baking soda is an effective "scrubbing" detergent and white vinegar works wonderfully for most kitchen cleaning (countertops, refrigerator, sinks, etc.). Why even keep "normal" dangerous chemicals in your home when non-toxic solutions are so easy and available?

✳ Consider buying a high-quality air filter for your home, and keep ample live plants in each room of your house. Palms, ferns, and English ivy are some of the most toxin absorbing plants around and they'll also oxygenate your air supply. A general recommendation is one plant per 150 square feet and to pay particular attention to your bedroom and other rooms you spend a great deal of time. It's also a good idea to just open your doors and windows regularly to air your home out.

✤ Avoid aluminum, Teflon® and stainless steel cookware. Stainless steel has often been considered safe, but it may also leach toxic metals into your foods. However, stainless steel is certainly better than either aluminum or Teflon, which are both highly toxic. To avoid toxic exposure with each heated meal, opt for glass or lead-free high heat glazed ceramic cookware instead. Ceramic can be one of the best options for heating food but not all ceramic is created equal, so make sure it's lead-free and high heat glazed. Ceramic from India, China, Mexico and Hong Kong or antique ceramic is suspect for having lead problems. Quality ceramic cookware can be found at www.ceramcor.com.

✤ Avoid using chemicals in your yard and around your home and look for environmentally friendly, non-toxic solutions instead. This will avoid polluting the soil around your home and the entire water supply from runoff. Orange oil is a great solution if you have termites or other pest problems. If you're up for it, it's a great idea to begin composting and nourishing the earth around your home too. Healthy soil is far less likely to have pest problems and you might also want to talk to your city or homeowner's association about doing the same thing on common grounds.

✤ Take care not to hold your cell phone next to your head— the same way you wouldn't put your head in a microwave. Using a headset that runs the sound through a tube of air, like the RF3 ENVi, is a good solution, as is using speakerphone. Many hands-free devices simply magnify the radiation to your head, so take care in purchasing.

You'll also want to keep your phone off as much as possible, especially if it's in your purse or pockets to avoid radiating other organs too. iPhones should be kept in airplane mode whenever possible because they release radiation even when they are off. You'll also want to take care when purchasing a phone and look for one with a low SAR rating, which is a measure of the radiation released. Under .5 is the best you can do and over 1 is on the high end. Also avoid using your phone with one bar or in metal cages, like your car. Both force the phone to work harder and can generate a hundred times more radiation.

✱ Do your best to avoid plastic bags and foods wrapped in plastic. Plastic easily leaches into plastic-wrapped foods and then finds its way inside of us causing hormonal and DNA problems. Be sure to also reuse and recycle any plastic you do use. Some health oriented grocery stores now recycle plastic bags which is great because plastic bags cost a penny to make but a quarter to recycle. Unfortunately, this means that many of them end up in the oceans forming the Great Atlantic and Pacific Garbage Patches—or what I call the cancers of the Earth.

✱ Enjoy plenty of sunlight each day to optimize your vitamin D levels. Vitamin D is a powerful hormone and many diseases are associated with low vitamin D levels—yet most of North America is chronically deficient. It's best to do thirty minutes to an hour of sun each day, with your skin exposed and without sunscreen.

Chapter 15

Wrapping Up!

I truly hope you find these methods highly effective and doable for *Cleaning Up!* your body. If I'd had these methods written out for me when I began cleansing, it would have taken *years* off the process. Had I known about the effects of toxicity and candida overgrowth earlier in life, I would have avoided years of suffering with so many health problems. I also would have spent a good chunk of my life leading a far more conscious life with benefits that will forever be unknown to me. My hope is that you will use these methods to end or prevent your own suffering, as I have done, and jump on the high-conciousness, elevated energy bandwagon too.

In any case, the methods in this book are the fastest and most effective methods for deep cleansing I've come across. And in my years of cleansing and experimenting, I've tried just about everything. Just about everything for me included many months of fasting (over the course of years), massive juicing, bottles of enzymes, enormous amounts of regular colon and liver cleansing, and dozens of different products and protocols. It also included an all raw, vegetable-only candida diet I followed for about a year and a half.

While I derived incredible benefits from doing all of this and got rid and improved of several health problems along the way (and many of these methods are in this program), it wasn't until I added the some of the key coffee combination enemas and massage techniques that large pockets of waste throughout my body and massive amounts of candida and filth *were even touched*.

Consuming large amounts of coconut oil, with these methods, takes detoxification to next level—and the soups and dressings are very easy ways to do it. If you've ever tried taking in so much coconut oil through other means, I'm sure you can appreciate this. The regular green drinks add another level of power, and it's compounded if you're using wild grass juices. Hydrogen peroxide skin cleansing provides even more power and it works to alkalize and remove problems from the outside in, whereas the baking soda enemas do the same thing from the inside out. Juice fasting with green juices and coconut oil mini-fasting are both powerful detoxification protocols too. And as long as you're not burnt out on coconut oil, I think coconut oil mini-fasting is actually very easy to do.

In any case, I really hope you now have the tools to get rid of most any health problem, no matter what the name, or how many people think it can't be done. Most people are likely to see improvements rather quickly using these methods. But most of us have been adding to our toxic burden, largely unknowingly, *for decades*—and it can take some time to correct your habits and really eliminate the majority of filth inside of you. However, it's one of the most worthwhile goals

I know. And when you experience living *without* all of this filth inside of you, you'll know why...

Health and energy are abundant. A spiritual connection is the norm. Your thoughts will be clearer, and problems more manageable. You can experience happiness and contentment—just about all of the time. Sages would call it an enlightened state, but many would call it an easier, more fulfilled, abundant life. Another miracle comes when we realize that we do have control and we can solve our health and weight problems permanently—and without drugs or surgery. For many people, it doesn't even take that long—especially when we look at the big picture. Many people also find that once they've cleaned up their bodies, they want healthier foods, so long-term dietary improvements come hand-in-hand.

But, when making lifestyle changes, remember to be kind to yourself. Just replace your poorer choices with better choices one step at a time. And if you happen to eat something on the poorer side, even while cleansing, don't let it get you down. Just move forward, with the next healthy step, one foot in front of the other. You'll get to where you're going.

And remember—cleansing is a journey, so enjoy yours! Also be sure to share your cleansing stories by e-mailing us through www.CleaningUpCleanse.com. We love hearing your experiences and cleansing successes! By sharing your cleansing successes with us, you also help us share them with others who might be facing the same problems—and would love to know about your experiences.

Appendix A

Getting Ready— What You'll Need

Equipment You'll Need

You don't need to invest in a lot of equipment to get started, but you will need a few things. With the exception of the enema bag, you may be able to borrow many of these things if you don't already have them and need to watch costs. A number of people doing the cleanse have also asked for affordable one-stop shopping, so I now offer many of these items on www.CleaningUpCleanse.com, including a cleansing starter pack and refill packs. The prices are often less than picking it all up yourself and it's delivered right to your door to save you from running all over town or paying shipping from multiple several websites. Plus, I include some e-mail based cleansing support with each kit purchased because it's not uncommon for people to have a question or two during the process. So, let's look at what you'll need...

Enema Bag ($10 and up)

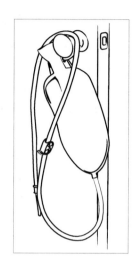

First, you'll need a two-quart or larger enema bag for self-administered enemas, and you'll needed get the reusable kind, as opposed to the single-use chemical kind. Enema bags are becoming hard to find locally and due to increasing costs, some brands have downgraded their quality. So, sometimes they're available at drugstores, but often their quality leaves a lot to be desired, and some drugstores carry them but many don't. Cara® offers a good two-quart enema bag and it's often available at Wal-Mart, but you'll need to ask for it in the pharmacy. A two-quart bag is a half gallon.

Glass or Ceramic Pot ($40 and up)

A glass or ceramic pot is used to prepare the coffee for the enemas, steaming veggies, and heating water for teas and soups. A large ceramic skillet is ideal for the vegetable sautés and I'm not sure they make large glass skillets. If you don't already have non-toxic cookware, you should purchase some for your ongoing heating needs too. Stainless steel is the next best option behind glass or ceramic and if budget is an issue and that's what you have, it's okay to use in this program.

Aluminum and Teflon are common cookware materials, but they leach toxic matter into your food while it's being heated and you don't want to put these materials in your body while cleansing—or ever. So, aluminum or Teflon should never be used and if you're having trouble finding glass or ceramic cookware, try www.shopworldkitchen.com/visions or www.ceramcor.com. See p. 165 for more on ceramic cookware.

Blender ($80 and up)

A blender is used to make the blended juices, soups, dressings, psyllium and baking soda drinks, and some of the herbal infusion enemas. Actually, a blender is key to making sure you're deliciously well fed during this program, and hopefully after too. The Oster® Fusion is a good quality affordable blender and the VitaMix® 5200 is a top-of-the-line blender that's really unmatched. If you're going to get into the healthy living lifestyle or are regularly preparing blended meals for more than one, I'd recommend a VitaMix, if the cost isn't prohibitive.

Glass Jugs ($5 each)

You'll need glass jugs to hold your enema solutions after they've been prepared and before they're put into the enema bag. A few half-gallon or one-gallon jugs are ideal and your containers should hold at least two gallons in all.

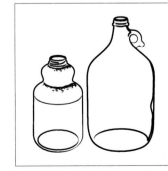

Large glass apple juice containers are ideal, but they are becoming harder to find. The best place to look is in health-oriented grocery stores, as most conventional stores now sell juice only in plastic.

Mesh Strainer ($15 and up)

A mesh strainer is used to strain the coffee and vegetable solids from the liquids for your enemas. It's also used for rinsing your nuts and seeds and for preparing nut milks. A medium-sized one is perfect.

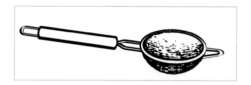

Hard Massage Ball ($20)

A hard massage ball is used with the massage techniques during the enemas. The ball helps loosen toxins in hard-to-reach places, especially in the back and shoulders. Massage balls can be found online at www.omnimassage.com.

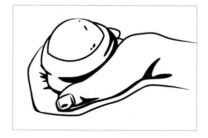

Optional Equipment

Different people will be willing and able to make different investments in cleansing, and I've written *The Cleaning Up! Cleanse* to be as simple and doable as possible, including financially. However, if you'd like to invest in the effectiveness and simplicity of your cleanse, these products are excellent ways to do it.

Juicer

There are a number of different juicers out there, and I recommend doing your homework to determine which is best for you. Generally speaking, they come in two categories: centrifugal and masticating. Centrifugal juicers are less expensive and easier to use and clean. They do, however, spin the juice, which destroys some of the vitamins and enzymes. But, if you won't juice unless it's easy, a centrifugal juicer may be your best bet.

Masticating juicers can be more expensive, as well as more difficult to use and clean. But, they produce more healthful juice by preserving more of the vitamins and enzymes. This is especially true with slow-speed masticating juicers. The Green Power Kempo, Green Star®, Twin Health®, and Samson® Ultra juicers are all good masticating juicers.

I've found that the Champion® juicer, a high-speed masticating juicer, produces a nice combination of ease and quality of juice. Because it's a high-speed juicer, you lose some of the enzymes, but not nearly as many as with a centrifugal juicer. Yet the Champion is relatively easy to use and clean, which I definitely appreciate. The only drawback is that it doesn't juice greens very efficiently. Breville's® Juice Fountain juicers are quality, affordable centrifugal juicers. The Hamilton Beach® HealthSmart Juicer is a great budget option.

Food Processor

A food processor that slices and grates, in addition to just chopping, can make preparing salads fast and simple. In fact, if you're short on time or regularly preparing meals for more than one, I'd definitely recommend a food processor. Nothing is easier than making hearty salads with the slicing tool. Cuisinart is well known for quality food processors.

Thermos

You'll need a stainless steel thermos® if you are preparing juice and need to transport it. Alternatively, you can use an empty glass juice container, and ideally keep your juice out of the light and refrigerated to preserve as many nutrients as possible.

Supplements to Have on Hand

You should find all of these in health food stores and I offer most of them in the kits on www.CleaningUpCleanse.com. However, due to current laws about what you can and can't say about the health benefits of substances if you sell them *and* what I say about coconut oil and baking soda, I don't offer these products. I simply prefer to tell you the truth about them. So, this is what you'll need...

Psyllium Husk Powder

Make sure you use *powdered* psyllium husk. Whole psyllium or seed isn't as effective.

✱ Good brand: Yerba Prima

Extra-virgin Coconut Oil

Make sure you're using coconut oil that is virgin or extra-virgin—as it's the only kind that's not processed, refined, or bleached. You'll want to start with at least thirty-two ounces, and you may want to invest in a gallon or more up front. The price of coconut oil drops substantially when you buy it in bulk and when you're using the high end of coconut oil on this program, you can easily use over a gallon each month.

Coconut oil can be found in both the food and supplement sections of most health-oriented grocery stores, however, it's often much less expensive to buy it in bulk on the Internet at www.tropicaltraditions.com or www.nutiva.com. In the U.S., Nutiva has the best prices and often offers free shipping when you purchase a gallon or more.

✷   Favorite brands: Nutiva®, Tropical Traditions®

Aluminum-free Baking Soda

Baking soda can be either naturally occurring or made from processing—and naturally occurring baking soda is preferred. Aluminum was once commonly added to baking soda as an anti-caking agent, but most companies are not longer using it. However, there may be some places in the world, like South America, where aluminum is still used. Just to be safe, I'd buy my baking soda from a health food store, and you can also buy it in bulk at reduced prices on the Internet. Bob's Red Mill is the only brand I'm familiar with that uses naturally occurring baking soda, and if you're going to be cleansing thoroughly, a 25 pound bag is not too much. Also, be sure you're using baking soda, and not baking powder! www.bobsredmill.com/baking-soda.html

✷   Favorite brand: Bob's Red Mill®

Probiotics

Choose a probiotic with at least five billion microorganisms and high amounts of acidophilus and bifidum strains. Ten to twenty-five billion microorganisms are recommended as a serving on this program, but more is fine too. Because most of us are lacking in this department, within reason, the more the better! Replenishing the healthy bacteria in your colon is important, so use only quality probiotics.

- Favorite brands: Renew Life® (Ultimate Flora Critical Care 50 Billion™), Nutrition Now® (PB8®), Renew Life® (FloraMore™), Mercola Premium Select (Complete Probiotics)

Stevia

Stevia is used as an herbal sweetener in many of the drinks and recipes. I've found it can really be a lifesaver when cleansing by making your drinks sweet and delicious and by eliminating sweet cravings. Plus, you need only a small amount.

- Favorite brand: Kal®

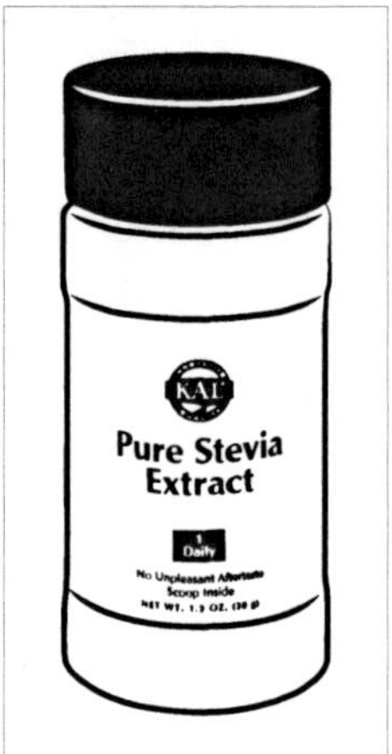

If you've tried stevia before and didn't like it, make sure you try the *powdered* Kal brand. I believe it's far and away the best-tasting brand on the market. Most people love the taste of this brand, even if they come to me saying, "I don't like stevia." Kal's liquid brand is, I think, the second best tasting brand on the market. Stevia is found in the supplement section of health food stores and if a store near you isn't carrying it, you can ask them to order it for you.

Cost of Supplements

On average, the supplements will between run $120 and $200 per month and the difference largely depends on the brands purchased and the amount of coconut oil and probiotics used. Coconut oil, in particular, can vary widely in cost, depending on where you purchase it. If you need to cut costs, you can use the coconut oil retention enemas less frequently and scale down your use of oral coconut oil too. It will just take longer for candida and toxicity elimination, but it's better to get started with what you can do.

Foods to Eat

It's best to use organic foods whenever possible. They may be more expensive, but they tastes better and they're a worthwhile investment in your health and well-being. So, just take a look at the foods and recipes, decide which look the best to you, then buy plenty. (Foods, Ch. 7 & Recipes, Appendix B)

* Lots of fresh vegetables and herbs for the salads, dressings, soups, vegetable wraps, sautés, and green juices
* Salad dressing ingredients (Recipes, pp. 185-187): lemon/lime, cold pressed olive oil, *organic naturally brewed* shoyu (soy sauce), organic miso, etc. Olive oil should be cold pressed and sold in dark bottles to prevent rancidity. For the same reason, you should also buy quality olive oil only in small amounts, and store it away from

sunlight. If you have olive oil in a clear container that's been around for a while, you should probably toss it and start over. Miso and shoyu should be organic to avoid GMO soy. Miso is always fermented and your shoyu also needs to be fermented, so only buy shoyu that's been "naturally brewed." If not, there's a chance that it's toxic, as *only* fermented soy is safe for consumption. Although, with the right brands, organic, fermented miso and shoyu are just fine. Good brand for shoyu: Ohsawa® Namu Shoyu (it's more affordable online)

* Coconut oil (also listed in the supplement section)
* Unrefined, un-ionized sea salt for minerals and flavor
* Raw, unpasteurized sauerkraut (Good brands: Gold Mine® and Bubbies®)
* Nori sheets. Raw nori is best, but personally, I think it tastes much better toasted. Nori is also more economical purchased in quantity. I'd also avoid seaweed from Japan.
* Herbal teas (avoiding chamomile or tea with chamomile in it; good brands: Traditional Medicinals® and Yogi®)
* Senna tea (optional)
* Raw nuts, beans, lentils, if you're consuming them

Ingredients for Enemas

* Organic, unflavored, caffeinated, ground coffee
* Aluminum-free baking soda—also listed above

* Greens like parsley, kale and spinach—ideally organic. Alternatively you can pick wild grasses; more in Appendix C. (Stage IV)
* Other herbs or foods in Chapter 8's coffee combination enema section (Stage IV)
* Coconut oil—also listed above (Stage V)

Purified Water

You'll need purified water for all of your drinking, food, and enema needs. If you're purchasing water, reverse osmosis or distilled water are your best bets, as most other processes don't remove the fluoride that's often in our water. Using fluoride-free water is important because fluoride is often the sole ingredient in rat poison and it has a mind-numbing effect on humans. Fluoride has also been associated with low IQ and brain damage in about a hundred studies, so it's not something you want to be drinking or using in enemas.

The water-vending machines located in front of grocery stores often use reverse osmosis and water can be purchased from them in bulk and at reduced prices. Alkaline water is great too, but these machines don't remove the fluoride so it's important that the water going into your machine is fluoride and contaminant-free first.

Whole house reverse osmosis units can run a couple thousand dollars, and if cost isn't an issue, I'd recommend one if your city fluoridates because unfortunately, fluoride is absorbed in the shower too. Undersink and countertop reverse osmosis units are also available for a few hundred dollars and can be great solutions for your drinking, cooking, and enema water needs. A water distiller is another option and if you're using distilled water, you can add some minerals back into it by stirring in a pinch of sea salt per gallon. If desired, you can also refrigerate your water to bring back some structure.

For home use, activated alumina filters are another reasonably priced option and with dual filters, they remove most of the fluoride. However, you'll need to combine them with other filters to remove the chlorine, pharmaceuticals, and other contaminants that are regularly in our water. Many companies that provide activated alumina filters online will also look up what's in your water, and help you make the best decisions about what you'll need.

In any case, on an average day, you'll need almost three gallons of water, and more if you're doing two enema sessions.

Appendix B

The Cleaning Up! Diet: Easy, Delicious, & Filling Meals

Simple, Delicious Filling Salads

The key to preparing delicious and filling salads lies in the uncommon. Lettuce, which isn't very filling, makes up 90 percent of most salads. But, if you skip the lettuce, or use it sparingly, and fill your bowl with lots of your favorite bulkier veggies, you won't be hungry shortly after eating. Salads made this way are also delicious, and you can vary them easily so your meals don't get redundant.

With all of your foods, organic is the way to go, but it's essential that corn, soybeans, or products made from them including miso, shoyu, or tamari are organic to avoid unlabeled genetically modified foods. Your foods should also be fresh, and not canned or frozen.

There are thousands of wonderful salad combinations out there using this "no lettuce" philosophy. So, use any below, or make up some using your favorite veggies. Making the whole salad by hand often takes just a few minutes, and with a food processor it'll be even faster. Just cut up your avocados by hand, though. Also, vegetable sizes vary, so feel free to adjust the quantities used. This is true with all of the recipes in this book, and you also don't need to be exacting with the proportions. In fact, once you get the hang of it, measuring isn't even needed.

Simple Salads—Just Dice Everything:

✱ ⅛ red cabbage, 1 avocado, ½ cucumber, 2 sticks celery, 1 tomato

✱ 1 tomato, 1 carrot, ¼ red cabbage, 1 avocado

✱ 2 tomatoes, 1 carrot, ½ cucumber, ⅛ red onion, 1 avocado

✱ 1 cucumber, 1 avocado, ⅛ red onion, handful of sprouts, handful of spinach, 1 tomato

✱ 2 tomatoes, handful of steamed green beans, handful of sunflower sprouts, handful of mung bean sprouts; 1 shaved ear of organic corn if you're candida-free

✱ ¼ green cabbage, handful of cilantro, ⅛ white onion, 1 avocado mashed with juice of 1 lime, alfalfa sprouts

✱ 1 avocado, handful of parsley, handful of cilantro, 1 tomato, ½ cucumber, 1 green onion

✱ 1 cup steamed broccoli, 1 cup cherry tomatoes, ½ cup steamed peas, 1 handful spinach

✱ 1 handful spinach, 1 carrot, ½ cucumber, 1 tomato

�֍ 1 red pepper, 1 cucumber, handful of cilantro, 1 avocado, ½ cup shiitake or portobello mushrooms

✖ 1 handful spinach, 1 avocado, 1 tomato, ⅛ sliced red
onion, ½ cup shiitake or portobello mushrooms

✖ 1 handful spinach, 2 leaves kale (de-stemmed), 1
avocado, 2 sticks celery

Salad Dressings

I've always believed that the dressing makes the salad, and
here are a number of simple, delicious dressings that don't
aggravate candida. Each of these has a different flavor too,
so by rotating them you can add tremendous variety to your
meals. Best of all, they only take a couple minutes to prepare,
so find your favorites and enjoy.

Blended Salad Dressings

These recipes are delicious, and personally, my favorites. Just
use the base ingredients, then add two or three additional
ingredients and blend. Some of the best use tomato or avocado, and if your dressing still needs a little something, try
adding a little organic shoyu too. These recipes are also easy
to double, or quadruple, and they do well covered and refrigerated for a day. However, if you're using coconut oil and
refrigerating it, it may harden, so just add a little hot water
before use, to melt the oil. These dressings are also easy to
bring with you, with veggies, for a snack or you can make
enough for a few meals at one time, for ease in preparation.

Base ingredients:

✷ 2 tbs warm coconut oil or cold pressed olive oil

✷ Juice of 1 lemons or 2 limes (if you're using fruit, the juice of an orange or a ½ grapefruit is good too)

✷ Sea salt to taste

Additional ingredients:

✷ ½ - 1 tomato

✷ ½ - 1 avocado

✷ 1 small handful of spinach

✷ ⅛ small onion (red or white)

✷ 1 ½ inch ginger

✷ 1 small handful of cilantro

✷ ⅛ tsp cayenne pepper

✷ 2 - 3 cloves garlic

✷ 1 tsp organic miso

✷ Fresh herbs, including oregano, thyme, cumin, basil, rosemary or sage

If you're using nuts, you can add a small handful of raw, probiotic soaked cashews, sesame seeds or brazil nuts—all are delicious. Almonds are also good, but not recommended for candida cleansing. (Soaking nuts p. 221-222) By adding more nuts, you can also make a dip for your veggies. Just add water to blend, if needed. If you're not using tomato or avocado, you'll also want to add a few tablespoons of water to cut the strength. You may also need to lightly warm your coconut oil in a saucepan if it's solid. With these, I use lots of dressing and have my salads in a big bowl, with a spoon, so I can scoop up a little dressing with each bite.

Easy Salad Dressings - Without a Blender

Because it's solid under 76 degrees, it often needs to be warmed before use. It's easy to warm on a stove, and as always, avoid the microwave.

* ✱ Warm (liquid) coconut oil, sea salt
* ✱ Warm (liquid) coconut oil, juice of a lemon, sea salt
* ✱ Warm (liquid) coconut oil, organic shoyu
* ✱ Warm (liquid) coconut oil, organic shoyu, juice of a lemon
* ✱ Lemon or lime juice, mashed avocado, sea salt
* ✱ Lemon or lime juice, mashed avocado, minced garlic
* ✱ Lemon juice, 1 tbs organic miso, 1 tbs cold pressed olive oil
* ✱ Lemon or lime juice, cold pressed olive oil, minced garlic
* ✱ Lime juice, cold pressed olive oil, sea salt
* ✱ Lemon or lime juice, chopped fresh herbs, sea salt (fresh oregano or mint are excellent)
* ✱ Lemon juice, sea salt
* ✱ Lime juice, seasoned sesame oil
* ✱ Cold pressed olive oil, sea salt, cayenne pepper (optional)
* ✱ Seasoned sesame oil, organic naturally-brewed shoyu, sea salt
* ✱ 2 tbs hummus, juice of 1 lime

Raw Soups with Coconut Oil

These coconut oil soups are a fabulous way to take in lots of coconut oil and they're delicious too. You can also add variety and create some even more interesting flavors by blending in any of the blended salad dressings on pp. 185-186, with or without the nuts. I strongly encourage this for some blow-your-mind tastes. These recipes are often large, meal-sized servings, but to make them as meal accompaniments, just half the recipes.

With these recipes, just heat the water so it's warm or hot, but not boiling, and then melt the coconut oil in it, if needed. With a VitaMix, you can skip this step and just blend long enough for it to become a little warm, so the oil melts. These soups aren't meant to be hot, or cooked, and even using hot water will just make them just slightly warm when blended—but it ensures the coconut oil will be liquid instead of solid for better flavor. Either way, just chop any veggies that need to be chopped and toss it all into your blender. Then blend, and enjoy. For variety you can also pour these soups over a bowl of chopped veggies and use them as a dressing for a half soup/half salad meal. Just bring down the soups sizes a little bit.

For extra enzymes and healthy bacteria, having these soups with a half cup of sauerkraut is great too—and while cleansing, this is best done regularly. Tomatoes and avocados make excellent bases for soups, so be sure to experiment and make up your own recipes, too!

Avocado Tomato Soup

✻ 1 avocado
✻ 2 tomatoes
✻ Juice of lemon or 2 limes
✻ ¼ cup warm or hot water
✻ 1-8 tbs coconut oil
✻ Season with sea salt
✻ Optional: 1 stick celery, handful of parsley, 2 cloves garlic, ⅛ onion or a little fresh sage and thyme

Tomato Garlic Soup

✻ 2 tomatoes
✻ 4 cloves garlic (you can substitute ¼ onion)
✻ Juice of 1 lemon
✻ 1-8 tbs coconut oil
✻ ¼ cup warm or hot water
✻ Sea salt to taste
✻ Optional: Add a couple dashes of organic shoyu for an Asian sensation. It's great with a little fresh sage and thyme too.

If you like it, indulge often for the benefits of raw garlic.

Green Guacamole Soup

* 2 avocados
* ½ small onion
* 1 collard green leaf or 3 leaves kale (de-stemmed)
* Juice of lemon or two
* ½ cup warm (not hot) water
* 1-8 tbs coconut oil
* Sea salt to taste
* ¼ - ½ tsp cayenne
* ½ tsp organic shoyu (optional)

Broccoli Soup

* 1 crown broccoli
* Juice of 2 lemons
* 1-8 tbs coconut oil
* 1 ½ cups warm or hot water
* Sea salt to taste

Asparagus Soup

* ½ bunch asparagus
* ½ tomato
* 2 cloves garlic
* 1-2 tbs coconut oil
* 1 cup warm or hot water
* ¼ tsp organic shoyu

Salsa Soup

✱ 2 tomatoes
✱ ¼ red onion
✱ Juice of 1 lemon
✱ Handful of spinach
✱ ¼ cup warm or hot water
✱ 1-8 tbs coconut oil
✱ Sea salt to taste

Kale Soup

✱ 8 leaves lacinato kale (also called dinosaur kale)
✱ Juice of 2 lemons
✱ 1-4 tbs coconut oil
✱ ½ cup warm (not hot) water
✱ Sea salt to taste

Spinach Soup

✱ 1 good sized head spinach
✱ Juice of two lemons
✱ 4 cloves garlic
✱ 1 ½ inch of ginger
✱ ½ tomato or 2 sticks of celery (optional)
✱ 1-4 tbs coconut oil
✱ ½ cup warm or hot water
✱ Sea salt to taste

Tomato and Herb Soup

* 2 tomatoes
* Juice of 1 lemon
* 1-8 tbs coconut oil
* ¼ cup warm or hot water
* Sea salt to taste
* Either fresh thyme, oregano, or basil

Crimini Mushroom Soup

* 1 cup crimini mushrooms
* 1 cup warm (not hot) water
* 3 tbs coconut oil
* Sea salt to taste
* Fresh thyme (optional)

Portobello Mushroom Soup

* 2 portobello mushrooms
* 1 cup warm (not hot) water
* 2 tbs coconut oil
* Sea salt to taste
* Fresh thyme (optional, but amazing)

Shiitake Mushroom Soup

* 1 cup shiitake mushrooms
* 2 tbs coconut oil
* ½ cup warm (not hot) water
* Sea salt to taste
* Fresh thyme (optional)
* Organic shoyu

Maitake Mushroom Soup

* 1 cup maitake mushrooms
* 3 tbs coconut oil
* 1 cup warm (not hot) water
* ¼ tsp organic shoyu

Mushroom and Tomato Soup

* 1 cup shiitake, button, king oyster, or maitake mushrooms
* 1 tomato
* 4 -5 tbs coconut oil
* 1-2 cloves garlic
* Fresh thyme
* 1 cup warm (not hot) water
* Sea salt to taste

Mushroom and Zucchini Soup

✴ 1 medium-sized *organic* zucchini, peeled
✴ 1 portobello mushroom
✴ 4 tbs coconut oil
✴ 1 cup warm (not hot) water
✴ Sea salt to taste
✴ Fresh thyme (optional)

Zucchini Soup

✴ 2 medium-sized *organic* zucchinis, peeled
✴ 4 tbs coconut oil
✴ 1 cup warm or hot water
✴ Sea salt to taste
✴ Fresh thyme (optional)

Yellow Crookneck Squash Soup

✴ 2 medium-sized *organic* crookneck squash, peeled
✴ 4 tbs coconut oil
✴ 1 cup warm or hot water
✴ Fresh ginger
✴ Fresh thyme
✴ Sea salt to taste

Mexican Squash Soup

* ✶ 2 medium-sized Mexican squash
* ✶ 2 tbs coconut oil
* ✶ 1 cup warm or hot water
* ✶ Sea salt to taste

More Coconut Oil Soups

The following soups have a bit of sugar or starch, so it's best to do them with some moderation and only with high concentrations of coconut oil. The squash soups are also filling, warming winter soups, and they're helpful if you're feeling cold or like you need more to eat. As with the other soups, just toss everything in your blender, blend, and enjoy. Depending on your blender, you may want to adjust the water amounts a little.

Carrot Soup

* ✶ 4 carrots
* ✶ 5 tbs coconut oil
* ✶ A little ginger (optional)
* ✶ 1 cup warm or hot water
* ✶ Sea salt to taste

Pepper Soup

- 2 red, yellow or orange peppers, de-seeded
- 5 tbs warm, liquid coconut oil
- A little ginger (optional)
- 1 cup warm or hot water
- Sea salt to taste

Acorn Squash Soup

- 1 ½ cups butternut squash, de-seeded and skinned
- 5 - 7 tbs coconut oil
- A little ginger
- 1 cup warm or hot water
- A little organic shoyu (optional)
- Sea salt to taste

Spaghetti Squash Soup

- 1 ½ cups spaghetti squash, de-seeded and skinned
- 5 - 7 tbs coconut oil
- A little ginger and the juice of a lemon (optional)
- 1 cup warm or hot water
- Sea salt to taste

Butternut Squash Soup

✱ 1 ½ cups butternut squash, de-seeded and skinned
✱ 5 - 7 tbs coconut oil
✱ A little ginger (optional)
✱ 1 cup warm or hot water
✱ Sea salt to taste

Pumpkin Soup

✱ 1 ½ cups pumpkin, de-seeded and skinned
✱ 5 - 7 tbs coconut oil
✱ A little ginger (optional)
✱ 1 cup warm or hot water
✱ Sea salt to taste

Guacamole

✱ 2-4 avocados, mashed
✱ 1 tomato, diced
✱ ¼ small (hot) green pepper, diced
✱ Juice of 2 limes
✱ 3-4 green onions, diced
✱ Sea salt to taste

Enjoy with a spoon, or on cabbage, celery, or sliced cucumbers.

Raw Vegetable Wraps

Many vegetables can also be enjoyed in nori wraps, and nori is detoxifying and a fabulous mineral source. Some great wrap ingredients include: cabbage, cucumber, mushrooms, spinach, kale, avocado, onion, sprouts, red or yellow peppers, skinny asparagus, and basil. Shiitake mushrooms are excellent in this. Just slice them all thinly.

Then, make a blended dressing with the juice of either half or one lemon, three tablespoons of liquid coconut or olive oil, two tablespoons of organic, naturally-brewed shoyu, and two or more of the optional blended dressing ingredients from the list on p. 186. Some great ones are garlic, cilantro, and ginger. Actually, a dressing with ginger, garlic, cayenne, and a little spinach or cilantro is excellent. Depending on the size, it may take three or more wraps to fill you up and this dressing generally makes enough for three wraps.

You can use a Sushi mat to help roll if you want, but I find it isn't needed. Just place your thinly sliced veggies in a line about an inch from the edge of the nori sheet that's closest to you, add a healthy dose of dressing, and then roll. Start rolling the side closest to you and roll away from you. Then, just tuck under the bottom (to seal it) and hold it at the bottom, so your veggies don't come tumbling out.

Nori is also an excellent source of natural iodine, but it's low in iodine, so most people would have to eat dozens of these each day to overdo it.

Herbal Mushrooms

Just turn over some portobello, crimini, or shiitake mushrooms, slice off the stem, sprinkle on some sea salt and top with a little very thinly sliced ginger or garlic. Alternatively, use a little fresh thyme, rosemary, or sage. Thyme, mushrooms and sea salt are absolutely amazing and this is a great way to regularly consume raw, healing herbs too.

Steamed Veggies

Chop your veggies and steam them over boiling water for ten minutes or until they're tender. When they're done, drizzle coconut or olive oil on top and enjoy with sea salt. Use lemon juice and organic shoyu too, for different flavors.

Some of my favorites:

* Broccoli
* Asparagus
* Green beans
* Spinach
* Carrots
* Spinach
* Peas

Sautéed Veggies

Sautéed veggies make a great dinner, or a wonderful lunch.

Chop and sauté as many of the veggies below that you like in coconut oil. But add greens, garlic, herbs, tomatoes, and other fast-cooking veggies toward the end.

* Cabbage
* Green beans
* Onions
* Tomato
* Broccoli
* Celery
* Eggplant
* Asparagus

* Spinach
* Ginger
* Green onions
* Leeks
* Bok choy
* Cilantro
* Parsley
* Garlic

When the veggies have finished cooking, season with any of the following:

* Sea salt
* Organic shoyu
* Sesame oil

* Miso
* Lime juice
* Lemon juice

Some of my favorite sautéed vegetables:

* ✱ Green beans, sea salt
* ✱ Green beans, garlic, sea salt
* ✱ Broccoli, sea salt
* ✱ Broccoli, garlic, sea salt
* ✱ Asparagus, cherry tomatoes, sea salt
* ✱ Red onions, garlic, tomatoes, sea salt
* ✱ Eggplant, garlic, sea salt
* ✱ Eggplant, garlic, parsley, sea salt
* ✱ Spinach, garlic, sea salt
* ✱ Broccoli, red onions, organic shoyu (add the shoyu just before it's finished cooking)
* ✱ White onion, bok choy, garlic, organic shoyu (add the shoyu just before it's finished cooking)

Beet Recipes, When Using Beets[*]

Tomato Beet Soup

* 2 large tomatoes
* ½ beet
* Juice of a lime

Blend with a half cup of water and flavor with sea salt.

Cucumber Tomato Beet Soup

* 1 large tomato
* ½ beet
* ½ cucumber
* Juice of 2 limes

Blend with a half cup of water; season with sea salt.

Asian Tomato Beet Soup

* 2 large tomatoes
* ½ beet
* ½ lemon
* ¼ red onion
* ½ tsp organic miso
* ½ inch ginger

Blend with a half cup of water until smooth.

[*] More about using beets in Chapter 12.

Beet Salad

- ✱ ⅛ cabbage
- ✱ 1 beet
- ✱ 1 carrot
- ✱ 1 sliced green onion
- ✱ 2 ripe avocados
- ✱ Juice of 2 limes
- ✱ Sea salt to season
- ✱ ½ teaspoon fresh thyme (optional)

Toss the avocados into a blender, add 2 tbs of water, the juice of two limes, sea salt, and thyme, and blend to make a guacamole dressing. Then, just chop the rest of your veggies, pour the dressing on top and enjoy.

Fresh beets can also be added to any other salad, and you might also prefer them grated. Beets, it should be noted, taste much better when they're fresh. So, if you "don't like beets," it may be that you've never had fresh ones. If that's the case, farmer's markets can be your best bet.

Boiled Beets

Boil whole beets for 45 minutes, or until you can slide a knife through them. Then, slice and top with a little coconut or olive oil, and season with sea salt. For variety, top with chopped cilantro and green onions after cooking is complete.

Appendix C

Cleansing Recipes You'll Need

Baking Soda & Psyllium Drink

Simply blend:

- ✷ 2 rounded tsp psyllium husk powder
- ✷ 3 ½ - 4 cups purified water
- ✷ 1 level teaspoon aluminum-free baking soda
- ✷ Stevia to sweeten

You can stir this drink or blend it, but either way, drink it quickly after it's ready, so it doesn't develop a gel-like consistency. If it does, add more water, stir some more, and then drink quickly. Also, rinse your blender well after use to avoid a hard to clean mess. If you're doing fruit and no longer using baking soda, you can also blend your psyllium with water, stevia, and a couple frozen bananas. It's also a great way to keep psyllium in your diet long term.

Blended Green Juices & Liver Tonics

These blended drinks are easy to make, wonderful detoxifiers and excellent ways to add plenty of minerals to your diet. The green drinks are also great pick-me-ups if you're tired while cleansing and drinking them regularly helps keep you mineralized, hydrated, and full. Fresh dandelion is a powerful liver tonic and you can add some in whenever you want to give your liver a little extra love. If you happen to be picking your own dandelion (from a non-fertilized or sprayed area), the younger plants are best and wash and use the root too; the root is actually the most powerful part of the plant. Feel free to also make up our own green drink recipes; these are just a few that I enjoy. And with any of these, just toss it all into a blender and blend. Then, drink with the chunks or strain them out—they're delicious either way!

Sweet Green Licorice

* 1 cup spinach
* ½ cup fennel
* 3-6 fresh dandelion leaves (optional, for liver tonic)
* 4 cups water
* Stevia to sweeten

If you like licorice, you'll love this!

Sweet Dark Greens

* ✱ ½ cup spinach
* ✱ ½ cup de-stemmed lacinato kale (also called dinosaur kale)
* ✱ 2 or 3 beet greens
* ✱ 3-6 fresh dandelion leaves (optional, for liver tonic)
* ✱ 4 cups water
* ✱ Stevia to taste

Sweet Greens

* ✱ ½ cup flat parsley
* ✱ 1 cup fennel
* ✱ ½ cup lacinato kale (also called dinosaur kale), de-stemmed
* ✱ 3-6 fresh dandelion leaves (optional, for liver tonic)
* ✱ 4 cups water
* ✱ Stevia to sweeten

Sweet Spinach

* ✱ 1 ½ cup spinach
* ✱ 3-6 fresh dandelion leaves (optional, for liver tonic)
* ✱ 4 cups water
* ✱ Stevia to sweeten

Sweet Spinach and Celery

* 1 cup spinach
* 2 sticks celery
* 3-6 fresh dandelion leaves (optional, for liver tonic)
* 4 cups water
* Stevia to sweeten

Sweet Beet Greens

* 1 cup fresh beet greens
* 3 cups water
* Stevia to sweeten

Wild Grass Drinks

If you're up for collecting it, you can also use wild grass in your green drinks and for the greens in your enemas. The benefit: grass is one of the most nutrient dense foods around and it's one of the most powerful detoxification greens available. Not only is grass incredibly rich in blood building chlorophyll, it also contains an essential fatty-acid that's hard to find elsewhere called conjugated linoleic acid (or CLA). Actually, because obtaining CLA from grass drinks isn't common, most people only get CLA secondhand, from eating animals that have been eating grass. But a better way to get it—go straight to the source: the grass.

So, let's talk about CLA and what it does. CLA builds strength and lean muscle, and it's a key reason that animals that feast on grass, like horses, are so lean, strong, and powerful. It's great for energy, enhancing metabolism, and dissolving excess fat while building muscle with exercise. CLA is also a potent cancer fighter and immune builder—in animals, even small amounts shrink tumors dramatically. And by juicing wild grass you'll be getting lots of CLA, and ideally you'll keep it in your diet regularly.

But, remember, you won't find CLA in parsley or spinach. In plant-based foods, it's predominately only in grass, although there's a little in mushrooms too. If you're concerned about keeping muscle mass on while cleansing, having wild grass drinks regularly is a great way to do it. If you have a cancer, solid lump, or tumor, I'd drink grass drinks regularly and also use them in your enemas. And believe it or not, grass drinks taste good too.

Interestingly, the absence of CLA might also be the reason that some people have problems on vegetarian or vegan diets over extended periods of time. Yet, by juicing grass, we get this powerful strength building nutrient without animal consumption—which I think is the best way to do it. Besides, we get far more CLA when we juice grass, rather than by obtaining it from animals. Grass is high in omega-3 fatty acids too.

More benefits: wild grasses are absolutely free and using them instead of store bought greens is an easy way to bring down the cost of your cleanse—while boosting the effectiveness of it.

Plus, understanding how to deliciously consume nutrient dense grasses can be a lifesaver in a food shortage situation.

So, to pick wild grass you'll need to know a few things. First, there are two broad categories of grass and only one type is used for consumption. Cereal grass tends have wider blades and blades of grass that are more flexible, and this is the kind that's used. Ornamental grass tend to have thinner blades and the grass isn't as flexible, or floppy, if you will. Ornamental grass isn't used for consumption. Then, younger grass, that hasn't yet gone to seed, is best.

The best places to find grass that hasn't been fertilized or sprayed is in areas that haven't been developed or manicured. Vacant lots, untouched hillsides, and the undeveloped areas between homes are often good places to look. Be sure and pick your grass away from car traffic too. Then, when you find some patches of grass, just tear off some leaves or bring scissors and cut as you go. If it's gone to seed, (you'll see the seeding at the top), just disregard that part as well as any brown parts and the roots too. You can gather enough for several days each time and then store it refrigerated in sealed baggies that the air has been pushed out of; stored this way, the grass will stay fresh up to a week.

Then, just before you're ready to use your grass, wash it in water. If you're blending it, blend about a cup with three cups of water, strain, and use stevia to sweeten. You can also blend grass with a lemon, grapefruit, or orange and stevia for some more sweet, delicious drinks, but strain before drinking.

Of course, you can also juice grass in a juicer or wheatgrass juicer that's specifically designed for juicing grass. Regular juicers and blenders work, but grass can be hard on them.

Fresh Low-sugar Juices - For your Juicer

Sweet Green Drinks

These green drinks are some of the healthiest drinks around, and with the stevia (and fennel), they're absolutely fabulous. Just use stevia to sweeten and make it delicious. Juicing a stick of fennel or chunk of the bulb will give it a delicious licorice taste too. If you like licorice, I highly recommend this. *With the addition of dandelion, any juice is a liver tonic, but just use 3-6 dandelion leaves per drink.

✳ Juice 5-6 sticks of celery or 1 cucumber with large amounts (up to 5 cups) of any combination of:

✳ Collard greens   ✳ Kale
✳ Romaine lettuce   ✳ Dandelion*
✳ Red leaf lettuce   ✳ Beet greens
✳ Spinach   ✳ Wild grass
✳ Parsley

Candida-killing Juices

These tomato and garlic drinks are delicious and an easy way to take in lots of raw garlic. Have them as often as you like, and the more the better! By adding a little sea salt, you can hardly taste the garlic. In addition, to get the maximum benefits from garlic, crush it and let it sit for ten minutes before use. Contact with air allows garlic's key germ-killing substance to fully activate.

✱ Juice 2-4 tomatoes, one lemon, and 5 cloves garlic
✱ Juice 2-4 tomatoes, one lemon, and ¼-½ onion

Tomato Drinks

✱ Juice 2-4 tomatoes with any of the following:

✱ Lettuce   ✱ Lemon
✱ Spinach   ✱ Lime
✱ Parsley   ✱ Cabbage
✱ Beet greens   ✱ Asparagus
✱ Sprouts   ✱ Celery
✱ Kale   ✱ Radishes
✱ 3-6 dandelion leaves   ✱ Onion
✱ Garlic   ✱ Wild grass
✱ Cucumber

✱ Use sea salt for flavor.

Celery Drinks

✼ Juice ½ - 1 stalk of celery with any of the following:

✼ Lettuce   ✼ Kale
✼ Spinach   ✼ 3-6 dandelion leaves
✼ Parsley   ✼ Onion
✼ Beet greens   ✼ Tomato
✼ Sprouts   ✼ Wild grass

Cucumber Drinks

✼ Juice 1-2 cucumbers with any of the following:

✼ Lettuce   ✼ 3-6 dandelion leaves
✼ Spinach   ✼ Onion
✼ Parsley   ✼ Celery
✼ Beet greens   ✼ Tomatoes
✼ Sprouts   ✼ Wild grass
✼ Kale

Lemon/Lime Drinks

✼ Juice 1 lemon or 2 limes

Add purified water and stevia to taste.

Beet Drinks*

✻ Juice 1 or 2 red beets with any of the following:

✻ Lettuce   ✻ 3 dandelion leaves
✻ Spinach   ✻ Cucumber
✻ Parsley   ✻ Celery
✻ Beet greens   ✻ Carrot or apple
✻ Kale   ✻ Wild grass

You can dilute these with water and sweeten with stevia, if desired. In any case, beet juice should always be diluted with at least half water, vegetable juice or apple juice, as opposed to drunk straight. Carrots and apples should be used only without candida problems or sugar sensitivities.

Sweet Blended Beet Juice*

✻ 1 whole red beet
✻ A few beet greens, a little spinach or some wild grass
✻ 3 cups water
✻ Stevia to sweeten
✻ 1 apple (optional)

Blend and enjoy.

---

* More about using beets in Chapter 12.

Cinnamon and Spice Tea

While this tea isn't officially in the cleanse, it's delicious and it's also anti-fungal, anti-parasitic, and anti-bacterial. If you add a little cayenne pepper, it adds a nice zip and becomes wonderful for the heart.

- 1 tsp dried cloves
- 2 sticks cinnamon
- 1 tsp dried allspice (optional)
- Touch of cayenne pepper (optional)
- 3-6 cups water
- Stevia to sweeten

Gently boil the cloves, cinnamon, and allspice for ten minutes, then strain, sweeten with stevia, and add a touch of cayenne pepper if you like. It's delicious and with all of the health benefits, why not consume it regularly, cleansing or not? This tea also keeps well refrigerated, so you can make large batches and enjoy it all week long. For extra anti-parasitic power, eat some of the cloves too, after they've been boiled.

Appendix D

Enema Preparation and Recipes

You'll want to prepare your enema solutions before you begin and bring them into the bathroom with you. Use your glass jugs to hold the solutions, and be sure never to put a hot solution into a plastic container.

Your solutions should be room temperature or warm, but not hot or cold. Cold can cause cramping, and hot can burn your insides. Especially with solutions using coffee, stick your finger in it first to make sure it's not too hot. Also, take care to use purified water, as tap water contains many contaminants you don't want to be putting into your body. (See p. 181 - 182 for more on the water to use, especially avoiding fluoride.)

One gallon of solution will make enough for two full 2-quart enema bags and in doing these enemas, you'll fill and release several times during each session.

Enema Recipes

Baking Soda Enema

✱ 3 level tablespoons aluminum-free baking soda
✱ Water to make 1 gallon of solution, total

Just combine and stir until the baking soda dissolves. In Stage I, double this recipe to make two gallons of solution. This recipe is also used to clean your colon before using coffee-based enemas.

Coffee Enema

✱ 4 tablespoons caffeinated coffee, ground
✱ Water to make 1 gallon of solution, total

Bring three cups of purified water and four tablespoons of unflavored, organic ground coffee to a boil in a glass or appropriate ceramic pot and let boil lightly for a couple of minutes. Then, strain the coffee liquids into your glass jug and dispose of the grounds. Now, add the remaining water to your coffee solution to cool it, and test it with your finger to make sure it's not too hot.

This will make enough coffee solution for a one-gallon coffee enema and you'll prepare the coffee portion of the other enemas using this recipe.

Coffee & Baking Soda Enema

✱ 6 level tablespoons aluminum-free baking soda
✱ 4 tablespoons caffeinated coffee, ground
✱ Water to make 1 gallon of solution, total

Prepare your coffee as described on the previous page. Then add your baking soda to your container, stir in some water to dissolve the baking soda, and finally add in the coffee liquids.

Coffee, Baking Soda & Greens Enema

✱ 4 tablespoons caffeinated coffee, ground
✱ The juice from greens, like wild grass, parsley, kale, or spinach (quantities Ch. 8)
✱ Other coffee combination foods or herbs from Ch. 8
✱ 4 - 6 level tablespoons aluminum-free baking soda
✱ Water to make 1 gallon of solution, total

Prepare the coffee and baking soda as described previously. Then, wash your vegetables, mushrooms, or herbs, and juice them or blend them with water and strain. Some of the smaller herbs and less juicy options are better blended with water and strained. Mushrooms and herbs are best fresh, but if they're dried, you can rehydrate them by soaking them in water for about a half hour. Then add more water, blend and strain. Seaweed will also need to be rehydrated in the same manner, but just for five minutes.

Either way, then just pour your vegetable and herbal liquids into your cooled coffee or coffee and baking soda for use. If you're going to retain this enema, however, leave out the baking soda.

With these, you can combine several of the foods or herbs into one enema, and of course, you won't need to be concerned about taste. You can do one, two, three or even four at a time, and if you're doing more rather than less, you'll want to use the lower ends of any ranges specified. With garlic and onion, you'll also want to make sure not to use too much, as it can become difficult to hold in the body for even six minutes.

Remember, you can do these with baking soda or drop the baking soda and just use the veggies, mushrooms, or herbs with coffee if you've had enough baking soda. You can also judge if you still need the baking soda by what you see coming out of you. If you see considerably more filth with the baking soda, and particularly if you see more white matter in your releases, I'd continue using it. If not, I'd phase it out or only use it on occasion—but for many people this will be deep into the detoxification process.

Coconut Oil Implant Enema

✱ ⅓ cup liquid coconut oil

Coconut oil is solid under 76 degrees and liquid over 76 degrees and if it's solid, you'll need to liquefy it by warming it over low heat (no microwaves please). Then, just transfer your oil into a glass container until you're ready to use it. Alternatively, you can pour a little hot coffee over your solid coconut oil to liquefy it. If you're warming the oil, be sure to check its temperature before use.

Appendix E

Easy, Delicious, Healthy Recipes— After You're Candida-free

After cleansing, a lot of people will want to help keep their bodies clean by upgrading their food choices. In this section are many easy, delicious recipes to help you do just that. These recipes are for after you're candida-free, however, if you're still cleansing and for whatever reasons are making occasional diversions from the diet, with the exception of the rice, fruit juices, or recipes using dates, agave, or honey, these are the best ways to do it.

Nuts

Nuts and seeds are great protein sources and they're wonderful for building lean muscle and rebuilding after deep cleansing. However, to benefit from nuts and seeds, they'll need to be raw and you'll need to soak them first to remove the enzyme inhibitors and activate the naturally occurring enzymes. Because nuts and seeds often have an invisible mold on them, which is detrimental to candida, you'll want to add just a little of a probiotic capsule to the water you're soaking them in too—which can help eat away at some of the mold. With this method we may not be able to remove all of it, but we can remove some. So, wash your nuts or seeds by massaging them under running water and then put them in a bowl covered with purified water and add a little bit of a probiotic capsule. Then, stir in the healthy bacteria and let them soak. After soaking, rinse your nuts or seeds thoroughly before consuming them or using them in any of the recipes on the next pages. Also, be sure not to let your nuts or seeds soak too long, and if you notice any film or coating on them, toss them and start over.

While your soaking times don't need to be exact, here are some guidelines to get you started:

✳ Almond, sesame, pumpkin, hazelnut: 8 hours or overnight.
✳ Brazil nuts, pecans, walnuts: 4 hours.

✳ Cashews, sunflower seeds: 2 hours.

✳ Macadamia, pine nut, pistachio and flax: 1 hour

If you're on a budget, sesame and sunflower seeds are generally very inexpensive. Your nuts and seeds can be eaten plain, or you can add a little sea salt to them. Some, like hazelnuts, almonds, cashew, and brazil nuts are great with stevia too. If you're not going to eat them right away, cover and refrigerate them, but don't keep them longer than two days. You can also use them in any of the recipes that follow.

Nut Milks

Nut milks are an easy delicious, protein-rich alternative to dairy, and they're great in many smoothies and dessert recipes. To make nut milks, use raw seeds or nuts (whichever kinds you like) and soak them in probiotic water as described on the previous page. Then, toss them into a blender, add about three times as much purified water, and blend until smooth.

When blended, just strain the liquids from the solids with a mesh strainer or a nut milk bag and enjoy right away or keep refrigerated for a few days. If you're drinking it later, stir in a bit of a probiotic capsule before refrigerating to make your nut milk a healthy bacteria drink. Your nut milks can be deliciously sweetened with stevia, a few pitted dates or organic honey—the later two should be re-blended in. My favorite is a few dates *and* a little bit of stevia.

You can eat the leftover nut or seed pulp straight with little sea salt or stevia, or use it make nut pâtés or nut cereals in the recipes that follow.

Nut Pâtés

After making a nut milk, you can take the remaining pulp and blend it with a few herbs and vegetables for a delicious protein-rich pâté. So, just take your remaining nut or seed pulp—or use whole soaked nuts or seeds instead—and toss it into a blender. To each cup of nuts, seeds, or pulp, add sea salt, the juice of a lemon or an orange, and two to four of the herbs or vegetables listed below. Then, add a little water to blend, and a little organic shoyu is often great too. After blending, your pâté should have a thickish texture and like the salad dressings, you can experiment and make up endless combinations.

* Sage   * Carrot
* Thyme   * Celery
* Onion   * Ginger
* Garlic   * Parsley
* Cilantro

While you're not limited to these nuts or seeds, cashews, sunflower seeds, almonds, pumpkin seeds and brazil nuts all do well in pâtés. After preparation, enjoy straight away or stir in some healthy bacteria and enjoy in the next few hours.

These are wonderful on portobello, crimini, or shiitake mushrooms, using the underside like a bread. Or have them on celery, cabbage leaves, cucumber slices, or just with a spoon. Here are some combinations to get you started. Just add a little water to blend and a tablespoon of olive oil can be added too.

Sunflower Seed, Carrot, and Herb Pâté

* ✻ 1 cup soaked sunflower seeds
* ✻ Juice of an orange
* ✻ 1 carrot
* ✻ A little fresh thyme and sage
* ✻ A little organic shoyu
* ✻ Sea salt to taste

Sunflower Seed and Celery Pâté

* ✻ 1 cup soaked sunflower seeds
* ✻ Juice of an orange
* ✻ 1 stick celery
* ✻ ½ red pepper (optional)
* ✻ A little organic shoyu
* ✻ Sea salt to taste

Cashew and Celery Pâté

* 1 cup soaked cashews
* Juice of an orange
* 1 stick celery
* A little onion (optional)
* Sea salt to taste

Cashew and Carrot Pâté

* 1 cup soaked cashews
* Juice of an orange
* 1 carrot
* 1 stick celery
* A little onion
* A little organic shoyu (optional)
* Sea salt to taste

Pumpkin Seed and Greens Pâté

* 1 cup soaked pumpkin seeds
* Juice of a lemon
* A little parsley
* A little cilantro
* A little organic shoyu
* Sea salt to taste

Pumpkin Seed and Mushroom Pâté

* 1 cup soaked pumpkin seeds
* Juice of a lemon
* A few mushrooms
* A little onion
* A little fresh thyme
* A little organic shoyu
* Sea salt to taste

Cashew and Herb Pâté

* 1 cup soaked cashews
* Juice of a lemon
* A little ginger
* A little onion
* A little fresh cilantro (optional)
* Sea salt to taste

Brazil Nut and Carrot Pâté

* 1 cup soaked brazil nuts
* Juice of a lemon
* 1 ½ carrots
* 2 cloves of garlic
* A little fresh cilantro
* A little organic shoyu
* Sea salt to taste

Sweet Breakfast Cereals

It can be challenging to find breakfast options that aren't loaded with sugar and often times GMOs too. Blended nuts make wonderful cereal substitutes and you can use the left-over pulp from your nut milks or whole probiotic soaked nuts or seeds. There are dozens of delicious nut and seed cereals to make and you can also combine your nuts however you like, but here are a few ideas to get you going.

Just blend everything, and if you like, top with fresh berries, sliced fruit, sliced dates, or a tablespoon or two of healthy chocolate sauce (p. 231). You can also blend any of these with a banana, fresh dates, and use water instead of a nut milk.

Sweet Flax Cereal

❋ ½ cup organic flax seeds
❋ ¼ cup nut milk
❋ Stevia to sweeten

Sweet Hazelnut Cereal

❋ ½ cup raw, soaked hazelnuts
❋ ¼ cup nut milk
❋ Stevia to taste

Sweet Sunflower Seed Cereal

* ½ cup raw, sunflower seeds
* ¼ cup nut milk
* 1 banana
* Stevia to taste

Sweet Almond Cereal

* ½ cup raw, soaked almonds
* ¼ cup nut milk
* Stevia to taste

Sweet Brazil Nut Cereal

* ½ cup raw, soaked brazil nuts
* ¼ cup nut milk
* Stevia to taste

Sweet Cashew Cereal

* ½ cup raw, soaked cashews
* ¼ cup nut milk
* 4 pitted dates
* Stevia to taste

Sweet Nut Desserts

Nut shakes, sweetened with stevia, are sweet, delicious and good source of protein. Believe it or not, you can even add whole greens, like raw spinach, to these drinks and they still taste fabulous! Try it, you'll see.

Sweet Nut Shake

- ✳ 3 cups nut milk
- ✳ 1 cup raw, soaked cashews, almonds, or hazelnuts
- ✳ 4 ice cubes (optional)
- ✳ Stevia to taste

If you want, add any one of the following:

- ✳ 3 tbs organic flax seeds
- ✳ ½ - 1 cup spinach or other greens
- ✳ 3 - 5 pitted dates

Just blend and enjoy!

Sweet Dessert Nuts

* 1 cup raw, soaked cashews, almonds, hazelnuts, or brazil nuts
* ½ tsp pure vanilla extract
* Sprinkle with stevia

Stir and enjoy! Alternatively, drizzle your nuts with a little organic honey and toss in some sliced, pitted dates too.

Chocolate Treats

Remember when you first heard that dark chocolate was good for you? Well, part of that information is true. Cacao is the seed of a fruit tree from which chocolate is made, and it's a rich source of antioxidants. Cacao also includes substances that raise endorphins and encourage the production of "bliss chemicals" in our brains that simulate the feeling of being in love, so cacao can be great if you're feeling a little blue. But, to really benefit from cacao, it needs to be raw (uncooked) and without dairy or sugar added. It's sold as "cacao" in health food stores and can also be found on the Internet.

Here are a few ways to enjoy raw chocolate and if you're like me, you'll find it a great indulgent treat. Chocolate, however, does contain caffeine, so use it in moderation.

Healthy Chocolate Sauce

* ¼ cup raw cacao, powdered
* 2 tbs olive oil or warm coconut oil
* ½ cup water or nut milk
* 1 banana
* 5 - 8 pitted medjool dates
* Stevia, organic honey, or agave to sweeten

Blend well and enjoy as a mouse or over any fruit you like. It's great over bananas, organic papaya or even watermelon. It's wonderful on soaked nuts too. Either way, it's a delicious fondue-type dessert, fun breakfast, great snack, or a healthy meal! It keeps covered and refrigerated for a couple of days.

Chocolate Nut Milk

* 1 cup of your favorite nut milk
* 2 tbs of the healthy chocolate sauce, above
* 3 ice cubes (optional)
* A little more stevia (optional)

Blend and enjoy.

Healthy Ice Creams

Frozen blended bananas make a wonderful ice cream sub-stitutes and best of all, it's a banana! If you're candida-free, indulge. With these, just toss everything into a blender, and blend until creamy. If desired, add a few dates in too.

Banana Ice Cream

* ✱ 2 frozen ripe bananas (peel before freezing)
* ✱ Water or nut milk to blend
* ✱ ½ cup of spinach (optional)
* ✱ Stevia to taste

Cashew Banana Ice Cream

* ✱ 2 frozen ripe bananas (peel before freezing)
* ✱ 2 tbs cashew butter
* ✱ Water or nut milk to blend
* ✱ Stevia to taste

Berry Ice Cream

* ✱ 2 frozen ripe bananas (peel before freezing)
* ✱ ½ cup fresh berries (use your favorites)
* ✱ Water or nut milk to blend
* ✱ Stevia to taste

Chocolate Ice Cream

* ❋ 2 frozen ripe bananas (peel before freezing)
* ❋ 1 tablespoon cacao nibs
* ❋ Water or nut milk to blend
* ❋ Stevia to taste

Frozen Fruit Drinks

Most fruit can be frozen and blended into delicious drinks, so find your favorites and enjoy. If you didn't freeze your fruit in advance, use fresh fruit and add in a couple of ice cubes. Enjoy these instead of processed, sugar-laden sweets, and you won't feel like you're missing a thing. They're also an easy snack or an excellent breakfast on summer mornings. Just blend and enjoy, and depending on your blender, you may need a little more or less water...

Pineapple Ice

* ❋ ¼ frozen pineapple (peel and cut before freezing)
* ❋ 1 cup water
* ❋ A touch of stevia (if desired)

Orange Ice

* ❋ 2 frozen oranges (peel and cut before freezing)
* ❋ 1 cup water
* ❋ A touch of stevia (if desired)

Grape Ice

* ✱ 2 cups frozen grapes
* ✱ 1 cup water
* ✱ A touch of stevia (if desired)

Watermelon Soup

* ✱ 2 cups frozen watermelon (cut and de-seeded)
* ✱ ½ banana
* ✱ 1 cup water
* ✱ A touch of stevia (if desired)

Fresh Fruit

Most fruit can be given a dessert-like sweetness by adding in a touch of stevia. Just sprinkle it on and enjoy. Strawberries are delicious with both stevia and ground cinnamon. Organic honey or agave can also be used.

Beans and Lentils

Beans and lentils are great protein sources and they're easy to prepare too. You'll just sauté some seasonings in coconut oil, toss in the beans or lentils with water, cover, let simmer, and come back later to check on them. When they're ready, enjoy a delicious, low-cost, high-protein meal.

Use any kind of bean you like: kidney, lentil, black, mung bean, and black-eyed pea are all good choices. It's also best to buy your beans dry, not canned, and they're easy to keep in bulk for regular preparation.

So, determine the cooking length and water proportions for the beans or lentils you're using. Generally it's about three cups of water per cup of beans, but do a quick Google search to find the cooking length and water proportions, if needed. Four cups of water per cup of beans often results in a soup-like consistency and can be quite delicious. Lentils are an excellent fast choice; green lentils take about 30 minutes, while red lentils are done in about 15 minutes. Soaking beans for four to twenty-four hours before cooking shortens the cooking time and can eliminate gas problems for those who have them. Just toss the beans into water the morning or the night before you'll use them.

So, first sauté any combination of the herb and chopped veggies on the next page in coconut oil (in the pot you'll use for cooking).

- ✳ Dried Cumin
- ✳ Fresh Sage
- ✳ Fresh Thyme
- ✳ Ginger

- ✳ Garlic
- ✳ Onion
- ✳ Celery

Then add your beans and water to the sauteed herbs and veggies (using caution when adding the water to the hot coconut oil), and bring to a boil. When boiling, cover the pot, reduce to a simmer, and cook for as long as the bean type requires. Check them occasionally to make sure your beans are covered in water while cooking. If they're not covered, just add some additional hot water.

When done, stir in some extra coconut oil to give it a thick, rich flavor, and some sea salt too. For different flavors and variety, you can also add in one or more of the following ingredients after cooking is complete:

- ✳ Ground turmeric
- ✳ Chopped tomato
- ✳ Chopped cilantro
- ✳ Chopped parsley
- ✳ Plain, organic yogurt
- ✳ Lemon or lime juice
- ✳ Cayenne pepper
- ✳ ½ cup of sauerkraut per serving

Varying your beans, veggies, and seasonings keeps your meals interesting, and if you use fresh sage, fresh thyme, and cumin liberally, it's hard to go wrong.

Rice Dishes

Rice is a staple around the world, but unfortunately most of it is nutrient-stripped white rice—or, worse "instant rice." For nutrition's sake, use brown or wild rice instead. Organic short grain brown is one of the best tasting, in my opinion.

So, first, you'll want to determine the appropriate water amount and cooking length for the rice you're using; generally it's two cups of water per cup of rice and about 50 minutes, but do a quick Internet search if needed. Then boil your water and when it's boiling, add your rice, a teaspoon of coconut oil, and a pinch of sea salt. Next, bring it back to a boil, cover, reduce the heat to a simmer, and let cook until done.

When your rice is done, top with some of these raw veggies (finely sliced) and add more coconut oil, if desired:

* Onion
* Tomatoes
* Parsley
* Cilantro

* Cucumber
* Kale
* Cabbage
* Mushrooms

You can use any of the vegetable wraps dressings (p. 190) as a sauce or any of these options:

* Sea salt
* Organic shoyu

* Sesame oil
* Miso

More Simple Salad Dressings

These dressings are pretty much the same as the ones in Appendix B, the only difference is that you'll use apple cider vinegar instead of lemon or lime. Just use the first three ingredients as a base, then add two or three of the additional ingredients and blend for a minute. These are for single servings, but they're easy to double, or quadruple, as needed. They're best with tomato, avocado, or a little extra water, and a little organic shoyu can also be added for extra flavor.

Base ingredients:

- ✳ 3 tbs cold pressed olive or liquid coconut oil
- ✳ 3 tbs apple cider vinegar
- ✳ Sea salt to taste

Additional ingredients:

- ✳ ½ - 1 tomato
- ✳ ½ - 1 avocado
- ✳ 1 small handful of spinach
- ✳ ¼ small onion (red or white)
- ✳ 1 ½ inch ginger
- ✳ 1 small handful of cilantro
- ✳ ⅛ tsp cayenne pepper
- ✳ 2 -3 cloves garlic
- ✳ 1 tsp organic miso
- ✳ Fresh herbs, including oregano, thyme, cumin, basil, rosemary, or sage

Fresh Squeezed Juice Recipes— with Natural Sugar

Carrot Drinks

✳ 4 - 6 carrots with any of the following:

✳ Lettuce
✳ Spinach
✳ Parsley
✳ Beet greens
✳ Wild grass
✳ Sprouts
✳ Kale
✳ 3-6 dandelion leaves

✳ Beet
✳ Celery
✳ Apple
✳ Cabbage
✳ Cucumber
✳ Garlic
✳ White onion

Apple Drinks

✳ 2 apples with any of the following:

✳ Lettuce
✳ Spinach
✳ Parsley
✳ Beet greens
✳ Wild grass
✳ ½ inch ginger
✳ Cabbage
✳ Oranges
✳ Grapefruit
✳ Pineapple

✳ Sprouts
✳ Kale
✳ 3-6 dandelion leaves
✳ Lemon
✳ Celery
✳ Cantaloupe
✳ Grapes
✳ Strawberries
✳ Blueberries

Orange Drinks

* 3 oranges with any of the following:

* Pear
* Lemon
* Blueberries
* Wild grass
* Strawberries
* Grapefruit
* Pineapple

Other Fruit Drinks

Any of these:

* ½ pineapple
* 1 cantaloupe
* 2 grapefruit
* 3 pears & 1 inch ginger
* ¼ watermelon

Baby Food

Making homemade baby food is so easy it's surprising more people don't do it to give their babies a healthy start with enzyme-rich fresh food instead of preservative-packed canned food. To make fresh baby food, just blend any fruit or vegetable well, adding enough water to make it creamy. If the vegetable is hard, like a carrot, just make sure it's blended thoroughly, without any chunks. With fruit, you can also add a tiny touch of stevia for extra sugar-free sweetness, and some fresh greens like spinach, parsley, or kale too. Below are just a few examples.

- ✱ 5 strawberries, water, blend
- ✱ 1 banana, water, blend
- ✱ ½ apple, water, blend
- ✱ ⅓ papaya, water, blend
- ✱ ⅓ cup steamed peas, water, blend
- ✱ 1 carrot, water, blend

Breinigsville, PA USA
05 April 2011
259164BV00003B/1/P